BEAUTY AND THE BEASTLY MARKET

TAMING UNCERTAINTIES IN MARKETING BEAUTY PRODUCTS

BILL KOSLOWE

Copyright 1998, Pinnacle Marketing Management. All rights reserved. No part of this book may be reproduced, stored in a retrieval system, or transmitted in any form or by any means—electronic, mechanical, photocopying, recording, or otherwise—without the prior written permission of the copyright owner.

Printed in the United States of America.

Library of Congress Card Catalog Number: 97-92289

10 9 8 7 6 5 4 3 2 1

ISBN 0-9659025-0-1

Pinnacle Marketing Management
Suite 465 Nationsbank Plaza
Winston-Salem, NC 27101-3915
Telephone: 336-856-8602

CONTENTS

Foreword: The Intrinsic Components of Beauty v
Acknowledgments ix
Introduction: How to Win the Game xv

PART I
Chapter 1 The Elements of Beauty Care Marketing 19
Chapter 2 Driving Forces in Beauty Care Marketing 25
Chapter 3 Requirements For Successfully Marketing Beauty Care Products 41
Chapter 4 Overview: The Women's Beauty Care Market 71
Chapter 5 Women's Beauty Care Segmentation 77

PART II THE BEAUTY CARE SUBSEGMENTS
Chapter 6 Marketing Cosmetics 95
Chapter 7 Marketing Skin Care 105
Chapter 8 Marketing Hair Care Products 119
Chapter 9 Marketing Women's Fragrances 137
Chapter 10 How to Bring a New Women's Facial Moisturizer to Market 143
Chapter 11 Phase II: Advertising and Product Development Process 157
Chapter 12 Phase III: Packaging and Product Development 163
Chapter 13 Phase IV: Market Introduction 169
Chapter 14 Men's Personal Care Market 173
Chapter 15 Conclusion 193

Notes 197
Index 209

Foreword

THE INTRINSIC COMPONENTS OF BEAUTY

BEAUTY—FASHION—ART—can we ever fully define these words? Truly they are not interchangeable and yet they are inexorably linked. What we consider to be beauty or fashion or art changes from culture to culture and time to time. There are no absolutes. Many people see beauty in the bust of Queen Nefretiti (1365 B.C.), the Venus de Milo (200 B.C.), or the Mona Lisa (1505 A.D.) but many people do not! Yet these three works of art are instantly recognizable. So when students ask me why the Mona Lisa is art, after all to them she is not beautiful, they have voiced the enigma of what is beauty and what is art. The reality is not all messages are beautiful, since art is a form of communication and, therefore, not all art is beautiful.

I will go on record in saying that Mona Lisa not only is art, but to me she is beautiful. And yet, what do people dislike about her? For one, she has no eyebrows; secondly, her forehead is very high. The fashion of the time was to pluck foreheads! Fashion is another concept that winds around beauty and art, for what is in fashion now seems (usually) beautiful to us. If concepts of beauty change from age to age and culture to culture, then what we think of as beautiful is truly what is in fashion. Philosopher George Santayana said, "For something to be fashionable is unfortunate, for it must ever afterward be 'old fashion'." If this were not true, there would be no beauty market to tame.

So—back to the original question—what is beauty? As stated before, beauty is not only culturally linked, but specific to a certain time. Which aging baby boomer wouldn't love for the robust proportions of Rubens' rosy "Three Graces" to be the current arbiter of taste. And yet there are a few things that most people will agree on: Youth and health are beautiful. Therefore, anything which aids the illusion of youth and health will be sought. Mystery and allure are beautiful, and are attainable at any age. Just think of those legendary beauties Kathryn Hepburn and Greta Garbo. Their beauty, allure, and mystery endure decade after decade. We can "ponder" whether Cindy Crawford or Claudia Schiffer are beautiful (and therefore enduring) or are they fashionable and therefore "doomed" to be "old fashioned." If the latter is true, will the beauty products they are associated with also become "outdated"?

What is it about this beauty label that so motivates people? Why work so hard to attain "beauty." There are inner motivators and external ones. Oscar Wilde once said, "One should be a work of art, or wear a work of art." A quote from Pablo Picasso said, "Art washes from the soul the dust of everyday life." If in this instance we substitute the word "beauty" for "art," then we have the lift that women get when they have made themselves feel beautiful. Think of the women who say that they put on makeup and "do" their hair even if they have no intention of seeing anyone or leaving the house. They do it for themselves, and they feel better for it. To look one's best boosts self-esteem and to have a bad "hair day" can sap energy.

On the external side, Edith Wharton, that great chronicler of early 20th century mores said, "A man's success is gauged by his wife's appearance, and who wants a dingy woman?" As offensive and degrading to women (and to some men) as this concept is, many men still feel this way, and trade in their wives of twenty or more years for newer models, in part to show the world how successful they are. So, a woman's thirst for beauty can be partially motivated by fear of becoming obsolete.

In the end, we can only be sure of one truth: beauty is a dynamic concept. It continually has changed through the decades and millenniums. The beauty marketer's challenge, therefore, is a formidable one. *After the product has been shipped to retail, after the advertising has been run, after the merchandising activities are completed, success will be measured one consumer at a time.* When all the individuals who believed in the message and product are added up, the marketer's success can be quantified. Traditionally, this is referred to as sales and share of market.

Beauty and the Beastly Market was written as a primer for taming the uncertainties in marketing beauty products.

DR. VIVIANA HOLMES

Acknowledgments

I HAVE BEEN FORTUNATE in my career to have worked with "world class" individuals as well as "world class" companies. Most of the folks listed below have spent a lot of time working with me on this book. It is as much theirs as it is mine. These people are not only colleagues, but friends. I not only learned the rules of marketing from them, but more importantly, the art of management and the tremendous degree of integrity that it takes to lead.

Dave Bluestein, former general manager of personal care for Colgate-Palmolive and president of North America for Duracell. Bluestein combines all the best qualities of leadership, particularly his ability to drive teams to "win" (i.e. he's one of those individuals that you don't mind going through a brick wall for). Bluestein not only understands the importance of strategy, but possesses the qualities to make disparate groups work "harmoniously" together. His skill in developing corporate strategy, coupled with an ability to motivate, are unbeatable qualities.

Joseph Campinell, former new products director for Chesebrough-Ponds, currently president and general manager of L'Oreal, USA. Campinell was the first marketing manager that I worked with in the world of beauty care. In 1977 he had a vision to take Chesebrough-Ponds into the hair care arena (it was strictly skin care at the time). Through his leadership and vision, he developed the Rave Hair Care Line. He did this by understanding the consumer gaps that existed in the marketplace and developing products against these "opportunity areas." Campinell's belief in "the consumer first" explains his success over the years.

Jay Friedland, president of Guideline Research, and Joel Benson, president of Joel Benson Associates. I have known these two individuals for twenty years. They have conducted consumer research for many of the prestige package goods and apparel marketing companies in the United States (i.e. Unilever, Colgate, Procter & Gamble, L'Oreal, Levi's, etc.). In my view, they are the two premier consumer insight specialists in this country. They understand "how to go to market" from the consumer's perspective and have provided invaluable support to myself and these companies over the years.

Jim Goldenberg, vice president, client services, Information Resources, Inc. (IRI). Information Resources has been an invaluable resource for both facts, and more importantly, hypothesis. IRI's scanner-based data across food, drug, and mass merchandiser retail outlets has provided not only the means for validating my conclusions, but it also provides a common way to view the beauty care market. I have worked closely with Goldenberg for five years and continue to be impressed by his knowledge, integrity, and client dedication.

Hampden (Bo) Keenan and Jane Martin. Keenan is a principal in the Renaissance Management Consulting Group, and Martin heads her own TQM firm. Keenan was the former vice president of human resources for Kayser-Roth, and Martin the vice president of total quality. These individuals have spent an inordinate amount of hours with *Beauty and the Beastly Market*. They have not only challenged the principles, but they have helped me become an author. I have learned from them that being an experienced marketer does not make you a writer. They helped make me a writer.

Betty Levine, president of Marketing Perceptions. Levine has served as a consultant for some of the leading image and consumer products companies in the United States (including Colgate, Unilever, Revlon, and Hiram Walker). Levine is the consummate qualitative researcher. She has a unique understanding of the human psyche, which has helped numerous Fortune 500 companies put forward product successes. From watching and listening to Levine probe the consumer, I have become a much more attuned marketer. Nobody better understands than Levine that the art of marketing is understanding subtleties.

George Lois, president of Lois/EJL. Lois is one of the most brilliant advertising men I have ever known (he'd be the first to agree with this statement). I have worked with Lois for nearly ten years and have to agree with his own quote "behind every great execution is an even more brilliant creative." Although I don't believe that even great advertising in and of itself can create a product, I do believe that without it, you can't succeed. Lois is a world class advertising man, and I have been fortunate to have seen him in action. He has been responsible for some of the most innovative advertising of the past quarter century (i.e. Lean Cuisine, Avis, Tommy Hilfiger, Minolta, and No nonsense to name only a few). He is a master at making a little expenditure go a long way (through the integration of different media—print, TV, outdoor, and advertorials).

Gary Malloch, former president of Chesebrough-Ponds Health & Beauty Aids Division, president of Faberge, and CEO of Kayser-Roth, and currently the executive vice president of Rexall-Sundown, Inc. Malloch is the consummate decision maker. His decisions are based on listening to the facts, taking a consensus "of the room," and then making a decision. These decisions are not always based on "majority rules," but carefully weighed against the hard facts and his experience. I have known and worked for

Malloch for nearly fifteen years and, in that time, he's been a hell of a lot more "right" than "wrong." Once his decisions are made, "it's on to the next issue." As I have discovered, there is no substitute for decision making.

Raulee Marcus, former executive vice president for Jafra Cosmetics (Division of Gillette), director of world wide personal care for Colgate-Palmolive, and executive vice president of marketing for Neutrogena. Marcus is one of the most strategically minded individuals I have ever come into contact with. Whether she is introducing a product in Topeka, Kansas; Nairobi, Kenya; or Paris, France, Marcus understands the operating environment. Her greatest asset is her ability to understand brand equities and how to mine them. I will always be grateful for the time that she has spent discussing the principles of *Beauty and the Beastly Market* with me. Her challenges to me have made for a significantly improved product.

Linda Nash, vice president of marketing for Clairol. Prior to joining Clairol, Nash was the executive vice president of marketing for Redken Hair Products and the group product manager for Chesebrough-Ponds Hair Care Businesses. Nash is one of the most intuitively bright marketers it has been my good fortune to have worked with. She has a sixth sense about what is right for the consumer when it comes to concept development. She marries that together with a tireless work ethic. From Nash, I learned not only the qualities that it takes to be creative but the necessity for continually taking the pulse of the consumer's mindset.

Christopher Nast, former vice president of sales and general manager of personal care for Chesebrough Ponds, former vice president of sales for Colgate-Palmolive's U.S. company, and currently president and chief operating officer of Rexall Sundown, Inc. Nast taught me what the other side of the fence is like; he was the first sales manager that I did an account call with (Pathmark in New Jersey as I recall). The true meaning of the marketing process comes to light when you sit in front of the buyer and sell your idea. Nast is not only the consummate salesman, he is a superb business professional.

Frank Oswald, former director of consumer insight for DuPont Fibers Division, and currently working on special projects. I have never met a person who was more highly thought of in an organization than Frank Oswald. For 42 years, Oswald led the effort to integrate consumer trends into DuPont's legware consciousness. His keen awareness of consumer dynamics helped forge pioneering partnership arrangements that included the vendor, manufacturer, and retailer. It has been a privilege to work with Frank and watch him help bring forth consumer products based on current lifestyle and attitudinal trends. Frank has never stopped being a student of consumer behavior.

Jim Santora, director of research for Unilever's Chesebrough-Ponds Health & Beauty Aids Products (Vaseline, Ponds, Intensive Care, Rave, Brut, Faberge); and Jim Figura, vice president of consumer insight for Colgate-Palmolive. The two "Jims" represent the best in what marketing research is suppose to be—understanding the consumer, defining business opportunities based on these "consumer insights," and detailing action recommendations based on these consumer findings. I have known and worked with these two individuals for more than twenty years. Their strength is their integrity, coupled with superb marketing skills and professional knowledge.

Bob Seelert, former vice chairman of General Foods, currently CEO for the newly formed Saatchi & Saatchi Group of advertising companies. I have known Seelert for nearly a quarter of a century. We first met when I was starting out as an assistant marketing research manager in the Maxwell House Division of General Foods and Seelert was the category manager of Instant Coffee. Seelert has tremendous abilities to take complex problems and find simple solutions that are both practical, strategic, and "right on." More importantly, he knows how to motivate and leads by example. He is an incredibly decent human being that has taught me the necessity of weighing business decisions against the cost of human resources.

Frank Stull, former chief financial officer of Maidenform, Kayser-Roth, and controller for Heinz. Being a marketer also means understanding the financial business environment. Working with Stull over the years has provided me with the insight necessary for creating marketing propositions that make financial sense.

David Vedehera, president Video Storyboards. Vedehera is one of the most astute communication specialists in the country. His company, Video Storyboards, has tested commercial executions for nearly every Fortune 500 company. His insight regarding communication vehicles and their ability to persuade, recall, and communicate broad strategies is second to none. I have worked with Dave on diverse categories (from panythose to vitamins) and have always been impressed by his ability to strengthen communication vehicles. His sage council also has immeasurably improved *Beauty and the Beastly Market*.

Lastly, I must single out four additional "parties": my wife, my kids, my company, and my dog.

- Shelley ("my wife"), has had the dubious distinction of watching me "niggle" every word. If not for her, there would be no footnotes or bibliography.
- Kerrie and Jessica ("my kids") managed to graduate from college without even being subjected to a rough draft. Seriously, their support for the past two years has been terrific.
- The Kayser-Roth Corporation (my company) has shown enormous patience in allowing me the freedom and support to write. **I would particularly like to thank Jed Holland, the vice president of marketing; Denise Landman, the vice president of women's department and specialty store**

marketing; **Ann Greeson, the director of marketing research; Steve Brinkey, the director of trade and consumer promotions; and Rae Mackall, the vice president of human resources.** I have received great encouragement and help from these individuals in developing this project. I will always be extremely grateful.

- Last, but certainly not least, I need to thank Sparky ("my dog"). She has had the unenviable task of keeping me company over the past eighteen months while writing and researching this book. (She's exhausted from trying to find a "clean" spot to sit in my office.)

Introduction

HOW TO WIN THE GAME

IN 1973, WHEN I RECEIVED MY MBA, the buzz word of the consumer products world was management science. Through systems and a systematic approach to problem solving, the art of package goods marketing, inclusive of beauty care products, could be "science-itized." Twenty-five years later, I can say without hesitation—consumer products marketing will never be a science! It is an art that can be mastered only through experience.

The marketing of beauty care products is the highest "art form" in personal care marketing. **It must be approached with a game mindset—similar to chess or Stratego—the winner takes all!** You can't win the game, however, if you don't understand the rules. The rules for marketing beauty care products were developed by the "masters" of this "art"— Calvin Klein, Colgate-Palmolive, Estee Lauder, Gillette, L'Oreal, Procter & Gamble, Revlon, and Unilever. Understanding how these companies think strategically and how they go about developing products and maintaining number one brand positionings year after year provides a "road map" for greatly enhancing your chances for success in personal care marketing.

Selling beauty care products is a fascinating process. Finding "just the right" positioning, marrying it to "just the right" element of functionality, and combining this with "just the right" proof to convince consumers it works is one of the most frustrating and engrossing problems in the world of package goods marketing. To a corporation, the payoff for success, however, can be tremendous.

Today, the beauty care industry in the United States alone tops $23 billion; worldwide it is a $66 billion business.[1] From the inception of an idea to the introduction of the product at retail, this marketing process truly takes on a life of its own. The minefields are enormous, which is why most product introductions fail.

No two marketing problems are ever quite the same, and no two companies approach marketing issues in the same way. I have been extremely fortunate to have spent my career with world class marketing organizations—from my early days at Chesebrough-Ponds to later experience with personal care companies such as Faberge and Colgate. I have partaken in more than fifty new product launches and have assessed nearly three thousand ideas for personal care products.

I wrote *Beauty and the Beastly Market* because there are no books that talk about the specifics of marketing beauty care products. There have been many books written about the elements of beauty care marketing, such as understanding demographic, socioeconomic, and lifestyle changes. And there have been books written about specific companies. But none has told the reader specifically "how to market" this category.

For purposes of this book, the beauty care market is defined as cosmetics, hair care, skin care, and fragrances. Although *Beauty and the Beastly Market* concentrates on marketing women's products in the United States, it also includes a "how to go to market" for men's products.

There is no such thing as a "cookbook" approach to marketing beauty products. However, there are certain "must have" strategies that significantly reduce the risk of failure. These strategies were developed by taking the collective best practices of the giants of beauty care marketing and marrying them to changes occurring in consumer lifestyles and socioeconomic conditions.

An important part of this book is devoted to generational marketing—understanding how to speak to adults in various lifestyle stages. It should be noted that this book stops at the year 2010 when 1996's oldest boomers will turn 62. Certainly life does not stop after this age. In fact, the over 62 population will number nearly 50 million by the year 2010. Nevertheless, the needs and wants of this more elderly market do change significantly. It is beyond the scope of this book to include an in-depth discussion on this segment.

The foreword by Dr. Viviana Holmes (a lifelong friend and a leading art historian from the University of Maryland) is important because it captures the elusive nature of beauty. It hones in on the most important dynamic—it is a *very* personal concept. All through the ages women have wanted to attain the elusive "beauty" label. Yet the concept of beauty is as fluid as an artist's brush—it means different things to different people.

This book is written as a practical guide for both the seasoned marketing practitioner as well as the new marketing manager—anyone who needs to get improved business results while reducing risks and improving organizational processes. The concepts and methods laid out are based on "real world" tools that form the successful marketer's framework for winning in the beauty care arena. It shows how to develop strong consumer based concepts, how to marry research and development with marketing to produce the products that deliver against those concepts, and how to deliver advertising with impact to targeted consumer segments that are large enough to deliver planned sales and profitability levels.

Beauty and the Beastly Market is your guide to taming the uncertainties in marketing beauty products.

Chapter 1

THE ELEMENTS OF BEAUTY CARE MARKETING

THE $23 BILLION U.S. BEAUTY CARE market has increased almost seventy percent since 1986.[1] Cosmetics is the largest segment with 32 percent, followed by fragrances (26 percent), hair care (23 percent), and skin care (19 percent). No category is smaller than $4 billion in sales.

There are at least twelve different sub-segments that comprise these four main categories of beauty care. For example, skin care

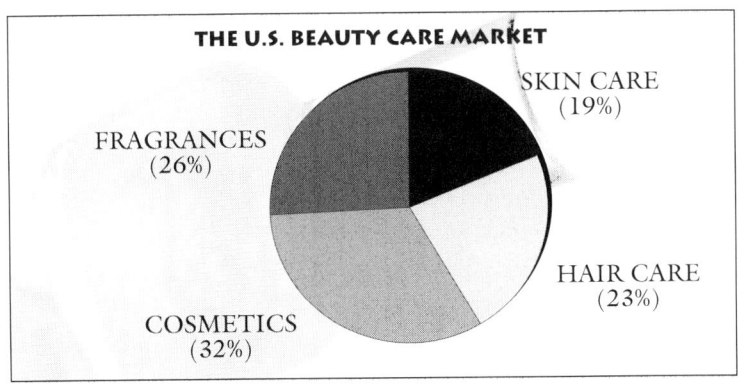

is really composed of hand and body lotions, facial moisturizers and cleansers, sun care, and bath and liquid cleanser products. Each has its own distinct marketing characteristics. To be able to market beauty care products successfully, it is imperative that each sub-segment be understood as a standalone entity.

WHAT MUST BEAUTY CARE MARKETERS DO TO SUCCEED?

There are three "musts" that dictate success in beauty care marketing. A successful marketer:

- Must have a focus on brands.
- Must understand the elements of brand positioning.
- Must be a student of consumer behavior.

FOCUS ON BRANDS

A constant theme throughout this book is the need to focus on branding. Brands will become even more important in the future, particularly for beauty care products. Why? **Brands shorten the purchase decision at retail, signify quality instantaneously, and provide confidence to both the consumer and retailer.**

This may sound like a contradiction since there has been explosive growth in retailer store brands across most categories over the past ten years. However, beauty care brands are one of the last bastions where the consumer places a higher price/value on a manufacturer's ability to provide a superior product. This is why "store brand" beauty care products have not been a major force in sales or share across most beauty care categories—store brands account for less than ten percent of beauty care retail sales in food, drug, and mass merchandiser outlets.[2] **Consumers will not "trade off" the real or perceived benefits beauty brands provide—they are not willing to risk potential failure if the store brand "doesn't work."**

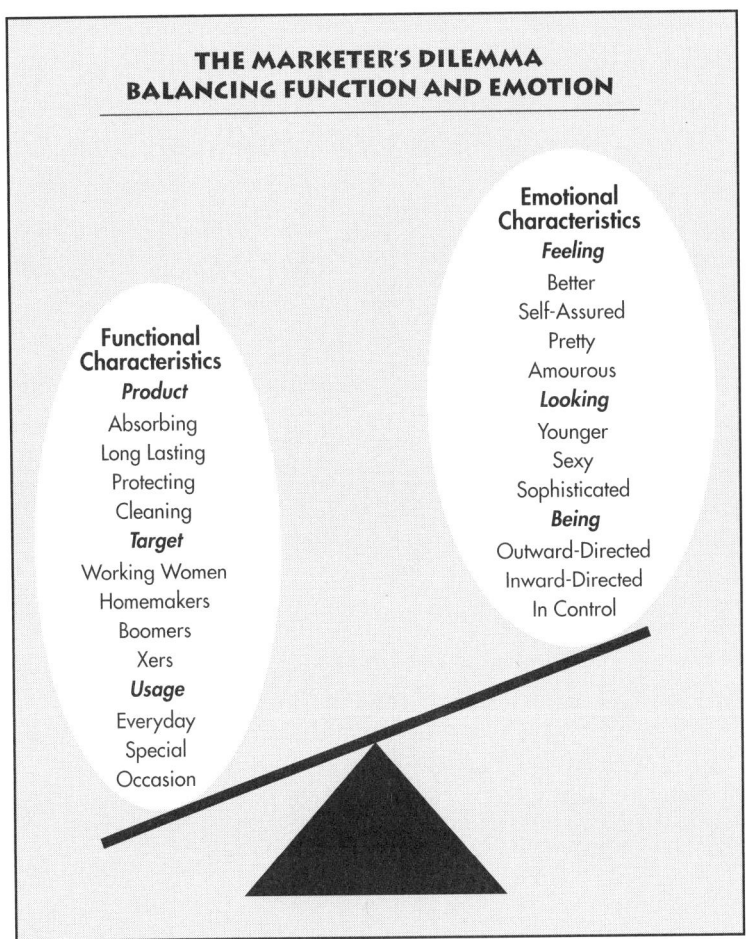

UNDERSTAND BRAND POSITIONING

To succeed, a brand *must* balance functional attributes with attributes based on feelings and aspirations. Brands must be emotionally integrated into the consumer's life.

This blending of product performance and emotional benefits is the essence of brand positioning! Learned marketers know that consumers are sensitivity to hype—there must be "real" added value for a brand to be successful. However, the "art" of "adding value" to brands is one of the most difficult elements of the marketing process. Mixing emotional payoffs (feeling sexy, being confident, etc.) and "real" product delivery (softer, smoother skin; clean hair; etc.) requires a fragile balancing act.

Charles Revson, the developer of modern day color cosmetics, understood the importance of appealing to both heart and mind better than any other marketer of his day. During the mid 1940s, Revlon (under Revson's ironclad leadership) began tying cosmetic color to fashion.[3] Each spring and fall new colors were announced, and Revson gave them attractive and provocative names such as Fatal Apple.[4] Andrew Tobias, Revson's biographer, summed up the strategy best: "Since it didn't cost any more to make a dark-red polish called Fatal Apple than to make plain, dark-red polish, and that one could be sold for six times the price of the other, this was not a bad strategy."[5]

Therefore, a constant theme throughout this book is the importance of brands and "brand name" both as a signature and as a product descriptor. **The lesson from Revson's success: Positioning is nine tenths of the law!**

HARNESSING THE POWER OF BRAND POSITIONING

There are three universal components that must be understood, managed, and balanced appropriately to develop product positioning that motivates consumers to buy: generational marketing, brand dynamics, and consumer mindset.

GENERATIONAL MARKETING

Understanding the principles of generational marketing is the cornerstone of the positioning process. In generational marketing, the marketer creates a picture of a consumer group by fusing together lifestyle, product needs, and more importantly, attitudinal wants of specific category users. In a broad sense, the first cut is to select who the key target is, such as Boomers or Generation Xers.

The differences between these two, both psychologically and economically, are huge. Specifically targeting to "generations" is by far the most important element for successfully positioning products.

Inherent in generational marketing is the need to refine the target (Boomer or Xer) to a specific beauty care consumer segment. Chapter 4 discusses the principal consumer segments of the beauty care market and how to market to them. For now, it is enough to say that there are four groups: Impressionists, Mature Stylists, Traditionalists, and Fundamentalists.

UNDERSTANDING WHY CONSUMERS BUY THE PRODUCTS THEY BUY

The second element of positioning is to understand the reasons consumers use specific beauty care products—what are the functional and emotional cues they receive and/or desire? It is important for marketers to refine product positionings so that their brand has at least one major point of difference versus the competition's brand. This difference is the vehicle for targeting the brand. This "single-minded" benefit approach is critical in developing motivating advertising and meaningful merchandising programs. (Chapters 6–9 discuss how to do this successfully.)

Although what a consumer requires of a product can change as a function of lifestyle and economic or socioeconomic shifts, there are still basic delivery requirements that have remained important throughout the past quarter century. For example, body lotions must moisturize, shampoos must clean the hair, and fragrances must have a scent. These fundamental "must haves" usually are referred to as "price of entry" requirements. **The art of "tweaking" or subtly changing these elements is at the heart of most successful brands' point of difference (this is usually referred to as the brand's USP or unique selling proposition).**

INTEGRATING BRANDS INTO CONSUMERS' LIFESTYLES

The third component in product positioning is the need to integrate brands into consumers' lifestyles. A classical definition of a "beauty" brand is the following: "A known name associated with a specific product or group of products carrying with it a sense or expectation of real and perceived values such as image, quality, cost, and confidence that you'll look good and feel even better."[6]

In my view, a brand is the embodiment of a marketer's ability to translate category needs and wants and lifestyle issues into a consumer business proposition. (Chapter 4 discusses this in depth.)

UNDERSTANDING THE CONSUMER

The essence of brand positioning is an understanding of the consumer mindset. Over and over again this book will stress that the only way to develop the "right" positioning is through a focus on consumers' desires, wants, and needs.

As the year 2000 approaches, it will be even more imperative to balance functional and emotional benefits. Beauty care companies face the challenge of trying to build businesses in increasingly mature and cluttered markets—this is not going to change in the future. The portal to success, therefore, will be to identify the most compelling consumer segments for both new and established businesses. Although this concept of "market segmentation" is old news, in the future a better term will be "market fragmentation"—selling products to smaller and more niche-oriented segments. Once these niche segments are found, the goal will be to ensure that they can provide maximum return on investment—profitable volume must be the end goal. (See Chapters 10–12 for details.)

24 *Beauty and the Beastly Market*

Chapter 2

DRIVING FORCES IN BEAUTY CARE MARKETING

THERE ARE THREE PRIMARY FORCES that drive beauty care marketing: product and consumer segment growth, socioeconomic/demographic/lifestyle trends, and future product needs. Successful marketers understand each and, more importantly, are able to project them into future use.

PRODUCT AND CONSUMER SEGMENT GROWTH

There are three primary avenues in beauty care marketing which can dictate a growth path:

- Overall category momentum, which is generally a function of favorable consumer lifestyle trends.
- Impact from acquisitions, mergers, and strategic alliances.
- Growth opportunities via market segmentation/fragmentation.

CATEGORY GROWTH TRENDS

Overall, it is reasonable to expect the U.S. beauty care market to be $29 billion by the year 2000. This equates to about a five percent per annum dollar growth rate or roughly $6 billion more than in 1995. Although all categories will expand in the years ahead, skin care will have the largest growth (+7% per annum) thanks to the aging population and, in particular, the surge in the growth of the 50+ group. Cosmetics also will benefit (although to a lesser extent than skin care) from this trend in the aging population (5 percent projected per annum rate). Hair care will follow at a 4 percent annual average and then fragrances at a 3 percent per year average.

Cosmetics, hair care, and fragrances will see less growth than skin care due to more casual lifestyles—in short, we will be "dressing up" less and needing these products less. (Chapter 3 discusses this phenomenon in more detail.) By the year 2000, the segments that comprise beauty care will have the following share levels:

BEAUTY CARE MARKET SEGMENTATION FORECAST

Category	Per Annum Growth Rate	1995 Dollar Share	2000 Dollar Share
Skin Care	7%	19%	22%
Cosmetics	5%	32%	32%
Hair Care	4%	23%	22%
Fragrances	3%	26%	24%

GROWTH THROUGH ACQUISITIONS, MERGERS, & STRATEGIC ALLIANCES

The biggest deal in 1995 in beauty care was the purchase of Maybelline by L'Oreal. This merger made L'Oreal the second largest cosmetics mass marketer in the United States. In 1995, the combined company did approximately $650 million in business (only $30 million less than the leader Procter & Gamble).[1]

The marriage of Maybelline and L'Oreal is an excellent example of why acquisitions, mergers, and strategic alliances will likely continue in beauty care.

- This acquisition significantly increased the distribution reach of L'Oreal. Maybelline nearly doubled the amount of mass market doors open to L'Oreal. (Maybelline was sold in 100,000 food, drug, and mass merchandiser stores versus about 50,000 for L'Oreal.)[2]
- Maybelline allowed L'Oreal a crack at the huge ethnic cosmetic market (projected to be more than $700 million dollars by 1997).[3] Maybelline owns Shades Of You, a pioneer in the mass ethnic market. It is estimated to have more than a thirty share of the mass market ethnic cosmetics business.[4]

The consensus of the top drug retailers, as well as Wall Street analysts, is that the Maybelline acquisition by L'Oreal will strengthen both companies. As one analyst said, "Maybelline is good at understanding the customer, right down to the shelf level. L'Oreal has the marketing expertise."[5] Retailers do not expect to see a "L'Orealization" of Maybelline or a "Maybellization" of L'Oreal.[6] **The cosmetic industry historically has been successful in terms of brands not only surviving acquisition, but actually benefiting as a result.**

Chesebrough-Ponds' stable of brands—Vaseline, Ponds, Rave—have exceeded category growth levels since its acquisition in 1986 by Unilever. This is a function of Unilever's infusion of both capital and international marketing expertise.

Industry analysts also point to Procter & Gamble with Max Factor and Cover Girl and Revlon with Almay as examples of acquisitions that have benefited companies and brands.[7]

Bottom line—companies can, and must, manage different brands successfully—even in the same categories.

Driving Forces in Beauty Care Marketing

GROWTH THROUGH CONSUMER FRAGMENTATION

The only way to market beauty care products successfully is through an understanding of the mega demographic, socioeconomic, and psychographic forces that will drive attitudes and purchasing habits in the future.

The beauty care market is reflective of general demographic changes, but equally important are pyschographic changes. Regardless of which beauty care product category marketers are talking to, they continually are faced with moving targets from both a demographic and pyschographic standpoint.

The difficulty in marketing to "moving targets" can be seen in the relatively poor hit rate of new product successes. Information Resources, Inc., the premier supplier of scanner-based data across all product categories sold in food, drug, and discount stores, reported that new products (whether they are line extensions of existing brands or really "new news") are being introduced at an ever increasing pace. In 1994 alone, 15,000 new item introductions went into food, drug, and discount stores.[8] However, more than seventy percent of the new brands failed and more than half of the line extensions failed.[9]

A key reason for this failure rate is that most packaged goods marketers have only given lip service to differentiating their products and messages along true demographic and psychographic dimensions. **Marketers must come to the realization that marketing fragmentation (marketing products to well-defined small segments) will be the key to success, if not survival.**

In essence, fragmentation is the "art" of taking a traditional market segment and breaking it down to even smaller groups of individuals who share common attitudes, demographics, and product usage characteristics.

The danger is taking this concept too far—marketing fragmentation easily can be confused with product proliferation. Product proliferation simply means an array of similar products all having the same benefit. Procter & Gamble virtually pioneered the concept of "fragmentation marketing" in the 1960s—but by the 1980s and through the mid-1990s this turned into product proliferation. (By 1994, there were thirty-one varieties of Head & Shoulders Shampoo and fifty-two varieties of Crest Toothpaste.[10])

The front cover of the September 9, 1996 issue of *Business Week* proclaimed: "Marketing—Make It Simple." This lead article extolled the virtues of Procter & Gamble in terms of the company pairing back SKUs (individual stock keeping units) as well as brands that were way past their prime. (Procter & Gamble has made a concerted effort to discard brands that were only marginal performers so that it can concentrate on its stable of market leaders.) The essence of this article was that "less is more" in terms of profits per stock keeping unit. Although no one can disagree with this concept (it's a pillar of prudent product management), it still doesn't negate the value of targeting specific niche segments. In fact, it validates this concept because it allows for more emphasis on "real" product differentiation. Procter & Gamble is merely going back to the strategy that made it the leader in virtually every field it entered—**real** market segmentation through **real** product differentiation to **really** distinct target consumers.

The art of successfully marketing to these distinct segments is contingent on understanding the mega-forces that will be driving beauty care marketing in the years ahead.

SOCIOECONOMIC/DEMOGRAPHIC/ LIFESTYLE TRENDS

Socioeconomic, demographic, and lifestyle trends point the way to marketing beauty care products in the future. These trends show a necessity to speak to the various "generations" of consumers; demonstrate the opportunity of rising family incomes; recognize the impact of an increasing number of women in the work force; and point to the potential for ethnic beauty care products.

GENERATIONAL MARKETING: BOOMERS VS. GENERATION XERS

Most marketers are still treating Boomers (those adults born between 1946–1964) as if they were one homogeneous group. The "oldest Boomers" (those that have just reached the ripe "young" age of 50) are not of the same mindset as those that have gone before them—or of young Boomers and Generation Xers who will follow them.

MARKETING TO OLDER BOOMERS

Older Boomers come with the attitude that "all things are possible."[11] Their whole experience is based on certainties:

- They were born into the boom economy of post-World War II, and so reaped the benefits of the "American Dream." In this era of stay-at-home Moms, Levit Town, Elvis, Barbie, and Hoola Hoops, all things were possible.
- Their rebellious, antiauthoritarian nature (nurtured in the 1960s and early 1970s) schooled them for how to "get theirs" in the materialistic 1980s.
- In the 1990s, this same individualistic spirit gave rise to the huge growth of entreprenuerialism.

These aging Boomers will be more "cool greaser than arthritic geezer."[12] They will continue to carry many of their trendy, somewhat extravagant tastes (learned in the decade of the 1980s) into "older age." Relaxed clothing, anti-aging skin creams, and whitening toothpastes will typify the growing influence of aging Boomers. In the year 2010, there will be 50 million Americans over 50 years of age.[13]

"This (older group) will be very much into beauty and is most likely to have cosmetic surgery. They want milder formulations, softer colors, and products that medicate *and* beautify," according to writer Iris Risendahl in *Drug Topics* magazine.[14] These will be

ADULT POPULATION SHIFTS[11]

	Boomers 31–49	Xers 19–30	Mature 50–62	Total
1995				
Millions People	78	45	31	154
Share of Total Population	29.5%	17.0%	11.7%	58.2%
Share of Adult Population	40.7%	23.4%	16.1%	80.2%
2010				
Millions People	72	47	50	169
Share of Total Population	25.4%	16.6%	17.7%	59.7%
Share of Adult Population	33.4%	21.9%	23.3%	78.6%
CHANGE				
Millions People	-7.6%	+4.4%	+61%	+10%
Share of Total Population	-4.1 Points	-0.4 Points	+7.0 Points	
Share of Adult Population	-7.3 Points	-1.5 Points	+7.2 Points	

people with attitudes much younger than their age. They will continue to be into fitness and have a greater trust in "the science" of cosmetics; anti-aging products must be based on scientific proof. **Therefore, it is likely that Boomers will become even more sophisticated consumers than they are today as well as more discriminating about the beauty care products they will use.** Skin moisturizers, cosmetics, and hair coloring products will benefit significantly from this trend.

MARKETING TO YOUNGER BOOMERS

Younger Boomers (early 30s to mid-40s) will differ significantly from the older Boomers. Younger Boomers come with a much more pragmatic approach to shopping.

- They already have adopted "value shopping habits" and feel the need to leverage their dollars. They plan ahead more and think more "strategically" in terms of finding the best price-value in the marketplace.

- These "strategies" already are characterized by consumers shopping nontraditional (or alternative) channels— Warehouse Clubs, SuperCenters, Factory Outlets, and Electronic Home Shopping (including both television and the Internet).

Despite these differences, there is one critical similarity that suggests that the message (or underlying positioning) could be similar for both younger and older Boomers: Although younger Boomers (like their older counterparts) are more comfortable with themselves than they were ten years ago, they also are consumed with maintaining their youth for as long as possible. This is not expected to change as younger Boomers age. **Hence, both younger and older Boomers could be reached with a promise of youth!** What must change, however, is the stimuli—the execution of that message. Since the year 2010 will have a representation of 72 million younger Boomers and 50 million older Boomers, this is reason enough for marketers to experiment with "getting it right."

MARKETING TO GENERATION XERS

The Generation X crowd (adults born between 1965–1976) has a whole different set of issues, wants, and needs. Their world is based on a combination of attitudes born from issues that were not major factors for the generations before them. Unfortunately, most of these border on negative associations—liberalized divorce, a stampede of women into the work force (which has made them the first generation of "latch-key kids"), corporate downsizing, sexual fear from the AIDS crisis, and the fight between church and state over legalized abortion. Given these negative dimensions, marketers have found that it is difficult to entice this group. Therefore, many have ignored Xers, preferring to focus on the more easily understood Boomers market.

While Xers (which number 45 million adults) are a substantially smaller group than Boomers, marketers have come to the conclusion that they are critical—if only because they will be moving into the "age brackets" of today's Boomers. As Douglas Copeland noted in his historic 1991 *Generation X* book, "for the shape of things to come, look not at the Boomers but at their successors." The real problem is: Tomorrow's Xers will not possess the same value structure as current Boomers.

Sneaker, electronic, and apparel manufacturers have had varying degrees of success with this segment; however, there are fewer successes in the beauty care arena (with obvious exceptions such as Calvin Klein's CK one cosmetics line). The reality is that marketers need to understand this group, because today's Xers account for more than twenty percent of the adult population and approximately thirty percent of the working age population.[15]

The economic and socioeconomic forecasts for the next decade do not indicate a significant change from today; so it appears likely that tomorrow's Xers will possess a similar set of values as today's Xers. Beauty care marketers must do a better job of communicating with this segment since they will represent 47 million adults by the year 2010.

Generation Xers are not only the heaviest users of beauty care products currently, but they are projected to continue to be the heaviest users of cosmetics, fragrances, and hair styling products. Even facial moisturizer usage, which is dominated by Boomers, is

BEAUTY CARE PRODUCT USAGE HEAVY PURCHASERS

	18–29	30–39	40–49
Hair Styling Product	46%	55%	60%
Blusher	43%	34%	23%
Lipstick/Gloss/Liner	42%	28%	29%
Foundation/Makeup	40%	28%	29%
Fragrance	38%	30%	31%
Eye Shadow	34%	33%	33%

Source: Karen Hoppe, "The Glamour Beauty Survey: Consumers Demanding Value, Convenience, Multiple Benefits," *Drug & Cosmetic Industry*, October 1995, Vol. 157. No. 4., p. 38.

SUN PROTECTION PRODUCTS USED REGULARLY (18-29 YEAR OLDS)	1985	1995
Lip/Eye sun protection	20%	43%
Makeup Base/Moisturizer with sun protection	NA	14%

Source: Karen Hoppe, "The Glamour Beauty Survey: Consumers Demanding Value, Convenience, Multiple Benefits," *Drug & Cosmetic Industry*, October 1995, Vol. 157. No. 4., p. 38.

expected to be high on their list (forty-five percent among Xers).[16, 17] Xers too show a high concern for aging.

Generation Xers also will be prime targets for preventative products.[18] Usage of lip, eye, and moisturizing products that contain "sun protective ingredients" have increased dramatically over the past decade among 18–29 year olds.[19] This trend is expected to continue.

RISING FAMILY INCOMES FROM DUAL WAGE EARNERS

With both husband and wife working, U.S. households are becoming wealthier. Sixty-one percent of households in 1995 had dual wage earners.[20] Dual income households will continue to increase in importance.

CIVILIAN WORK FORCE: 1970-2000	1970	1980	1990	2000
Total (MM)	83	107	125	142
Male	51	62	68	75
Female	32	46	57	67
Male: % Work Force	61%	57%	54%	53%
Female: % Work Force	39%	43%	46%	47%

Source: *115th Edition of The Statistical Abstract of the United States 1995*, p. 399.

Beauty and the Beastly Market

Median incomes are approaching $40,000, with about fifty percent of that income classified as discretionary.[21] Importantly, the average household size is 2.5, indicating that many in this group are still raising families and/or have their "20 something" Xer still living with them. (More than fifty percent of Xers are still living with their parents.[22])

Dual income households not only have women that are earning about the same or more than their mates, but they also are significantly better educated than any other generation in history—eighty percent graduated high school, while nearly forty percent have some college education.[23] **The impact of these higher income and better educated households has been an increased demand for higher-end beauty care products.** (Dual wage earners have an increased ability to pay more.)[24]

MARRIED WOMEN'S PARTICIPATION IN THE WORK FORCE			
1970	1980	1990	2000
40.5%	49.9%	58.4%	65.0%

Source: 115th Edition of *The Statistical Abstract of the United States 1995*, p. 405.

MORE WOMEN IN THE WORK FORCE

Today the civilian work force is nearly equally divided between men and women.[25] However, since 1970 the growth has been significantly stronger among women (35 million women compared to 24 million for men).[26]

The female work force of the future will be older and consist of more single women than today. Women are marrying later, and divorce is increasing. In addition, older/married women (45+) are going back to work in droves.[27] Given the age dynamics and diverse experiences of these women, targeting niche segments will be a necessity.

THE WOMEN'S MARKET SINGLEHOOD: A FORCE OF CHANGE				
	1970	1980	1990	2000
Average Age Married	20.6	21.8	24.0	26.0
Divorce Rate (%) (Women 30-54: After 1st Marriage)	NA	25	33	40
Working Married Women 45-64 (%)	51.3	54.2	65	78

Source: 115th Edition of *The Statistical Abstract of the United States 1995*, p. 103-405.

UNDERSTANDING ETHNICITY

Ethnic diversity is and will continue to have an impact on current and future marketing plans of beauty care manufacturers. In 1995, nearly twenty-eight percent of the adult population was not Caucasian.[28]

Over thirty percent of the U.S. population will be non-European or non-Caucasian by the year 2000. Overall, ethnic consumers want mainstream products and brands; but they must be able to also address special needs.[29] The ethnic market is expected to be in the $1 billion range by the year 2000 (versus $550 million in 1987).[30]

To be successful, companies must focus on the content in their advertising and marketing campaigns to reach these different cultural groups or "market fragments." Central to this theme is the need to acknowledge the differences among the cultures, but without reinforcing stereotypes.[31]

- Products that create a more professional appearance will be particularly important to both African-American and Hispanic women as an increasing number enter the business market.
- African-American and Hispanic women already use hair coloring products more than Caucasian women—this will continue in the future.

	GENERATIONAL ETHNICITY				
	TOTAL	WHITE	BLACK	HISPANIC	ASIAN
Boomers	100%	76	11	9	4
Xers	100%	70	13	13	4
Mature	100%	80	10	7	3

Source: Susan Mitchell, *The Official Guide to the Generations,* 1st Edition, Ithica, NY: New Strategist Publications, Inc., 1995.

➤ African-American men will want more products that treat "foliculitus" or razor bumps. (See Chapter 13.)

➤ Asian consumers will demand a broader range of skin tones. In the past, this segment with a yellow-to-pink skin undertone has been difficult to formulate for. This group includes not only Chinese and Japanese, but also the native peoples of North and South America.

FUTURE PRODUCT NEEDS

THE TYPES OF PRODUCTS THAT WILL BE NEEDED

Socioeconomic, demographic, and lifestyle factors will present beauty care manufacturers with marketing opportunities (as well as challenges); both therapeutic and cosmetic products will be needed. For example, **women who fill many roles (wife, mom, date, housekeeper, banker, chauffeur) will look to products that offer moments of relaxation, provide stimulation, promise to "speed the process," or allow for "mood differentiation."**

Beauty care products are "active" oriented. Consumers are intent on seeing performance, and they expect that claims are backed up by "scientific" testing results. Beyond basic functionality (doing what the manufacturer says it will do), beauty care products also increasingly appeal to an expanding range of related consumer preferences—natural based products, non-animal derivatives, sensitive skin, and nonirritating formulations.[32]

MARKETING TO CONSUMER FRAGMENTS: THE PITFALLS & HOW TO AVOID THEM

Research indicates that the future will present an even more complex marketplace; targeting principal market fragments will be more difficult. Although "new news" is essential in beauty care marketing, manufacturers must fight the urge to proliferate with line extensions that either water down the parent brand or do not perform up to consumer expectations. Otherwise, brand franchises will be seriously compromised. Therefore, continued emphasis placed on research and development will be critical for success. **Marketers must consistently challenge R&D from both a product ingredient and delivery system vantage point to produce distinctive new products.**

- R&D in skin care, hair care, and cosmetics product ingredients increasingly focuses on treatment and protection products that can be integrally linked with "science." **Products that can "speed the process" (healing, moisturizing, cleaning, anti-aging) or "make the process easier" (save time, expend less energy, etc.) will win in the marketplace.**
- A critical hot button in marketing beauty care products is to realize that it is an active, problem-solution business with an increasing tendency to emphasize therapeutic end-benefits. R&D is expected to play an even greater role in the future in the "go to market process." R&D not only will be involved in product formulation, but in development of image and message.

Successfully marketing beauty care products will require an even greater in-depth understanding of consumer attitudes and values in the years ahead. This inherently means paying even more attention to psychographics and socioeconomic shifts. These mega forces invariably will affect people's behavior as consumers.

Case Study
EXAMPLES OF CHANGING CONSUMER ATTITUDES

The focus-on-self that dominated the 1980s is still formidable in the beauty care arena, a category charged with a strong emotional component. However, the recession in the late 1980s and early 1990s, coupled with downsizing in corporate America, have caused significant modifications in purchasing and shopping habits. This has led to a renewed emphasis on the "price/value" equation. Opportunities will abound for products at both the upper and lower end of the pricing spectrum. Marketers' brands squeezed between these upper and lower ends will have a more difficult time; they must offer a strong reason for purchasing—or perish.

The fragrance market is ripe with examples of products that have faded away because they presented either relatively weak ideas with "middling price points" or reasonably good ideas, but with price points that were so high that they created a poor long-term price/value relationship.

In the 1980s, fragrance marketers introduced products that were takeoffs of popular themes. For example Carrington and Krystal were introduced as a man's and woman's fragrance. Both were based on characters on the popular Dynasty television show and sold at the high end of chain drug stores (approximately a $12 price point). When the show ran its course, guess what happened to the fragrances?

In the late 1980s and early 1990s, because of the inherent strength of the price/value equation, many of the upper tier fragrance brands began to decline. The popularity of knock-off designer fragrances rose. The first major successful knock-off entry was Primo, which explicitly said: "If you like Georgio, you'll love Primo." (And who wouldn't with Primo sporting a $7.50 price tag compared to more than $40 for Georgio cologne?) The lesson was clear; the image of these fragrances was not strong enough to withstand the onslaught of their less expensive imitations.

A strong conceptual idea (a.k.a. "The Big Idea") is critical for a product's success. Without this element, a product cannot have long-term business potential. However, the Big Idea also must be rooted in the "known" in terms of product usage behavior. **Products that look to change behavior generally will have a small chance of success.**

> For example, in the late 1970s we saw the introduction of "deo-colognes." These were allover body sprays (like Unilever's Impulse) that were extremely popular in Europe. Deo-colognes succeeded in Europe because usage of deodorants (particularly in the late 1970s) was significantly less than in the United States. In the U.S., consumers were not used to putting fragrance "all over their bodies." This was particularly true in the men's personal care market.

As the year 2000 approaches, there will be a new emphasis on traditionalism (the 1996 Republican and Democratic platforms confirm this) and a tempering of the desire for novelty, impulse buying, and expanding wardrobes (due to the overwhelming embrace of "casual dress"). These directions will cause even more fundamental changes in the way beauty care goods must be marketed in the future. Consumers will take a more selective approach to shopping—and yet they will have even more "shopping" alternatives. The remaining chapters in *Beauty and the Beastly Market* discuss how to increase your success rate in marketing these products.

Chapter 3

REQUIREMENTS FOR SUCCESSFULLY MARKETING BEAUTY CARE PRODUCTS

TO BE A SUCCESSFUL MARKETER of beauty care products requires commitment. There are seven required "must haves" to be considered a committed beauty care marketer:

- **Must** have strong, well-supported brand names.
- **Must** have commitment to developing value-added consumer products.
- **Must** have a well-defined advertising strategy that begins and ends with communicating the Big Idea.
- **Must** be committed to habitually "refreshing" established businesses.
- **Must** have a strategic financial plan that is continuously monitored.
- **Must** have a well-defined trade channel strategy.
- **Must** establish the "right" retail price points.

THE ROLE OF BRANDING IN BEAUTY CARE

There are no other consumer product categories that are as highly charged emotionally as beauty care. The reason is simple—few have the risk associated with them as beauty care does. For example, you can cover a "bad hair day" with a hat and hope no one sees it. However, a "bad face day" can mean more than discomfort; it can be devastating emotionally (particularly if it is caused by an allergic reaction that manifests itself physically).

Because of this emotional factor, consumers generally will not trade-off branded products for cheaper alternatives (with the exception of "knock-off designer" fragrances). It is for this reason that private label beauty care products account for less than ten percent of beauty care sales.[1]

MEGA-BRANDING AND PRODUCT LINE DIFFERENTIATION

Branded beauty care products provide the comfort level that is required by the consumer in order for her to purchase the item. Because of the importance of brand names in beauty care, it was one of the first categories to use mega-branding as a means of developing new products. Mega-branding is the art of taking a successful brand in one category and placing it across a number of different categories. Established brands such as Vaseline, Oil of Olay, Ponds, and Estee Lauder were able to penetrate new beauty care segments because of their proven product performance in other beauty care categories.

In 1995, Information Resources, Inc. completed a study that focused on 240 categories sold in food, drug, and mass merchandisers from 1991 to 1994. The survey covered nearly a thousand items. The objective was to define what were the most successful characteristics among the "winning" new products. Information Resources defined a "winning" new product as a brand achieving at least thirty percent distribution at the end of a two-year period and at least $15 million in sales. The results indicated that of the nearly three hundred "successful" new products only fourteen percent were entirely new brand names—eighty-six percent were extensions of successful, relatively well-known brand equities (or repositionings with a new twist to the product and name).[2]

There is little doubt that **mega-branding will continue to be a popular form for introducing products; it is cost efficient in terms of creating awareness, it saves money in terms of inducing trial, and the parent brand is already a "proven" money maker with the trade.** However, it also presents the most danger in terms of protecting core brand franchises. If the fit of the line extension is different from the parent and it is not perceived in a positive light by the consumer, it can have a disastrous effect on the original ("parent") brand.

A Case Study

COLGATE-PALMOLIVE FACIAL BAR SOAP

A classic example in the United States where line extending a brand had a devastating effect on the core franchise can be seen in the case of Palmolive Bar Soap. In the early 1960s, Palmolive Facial Bar Soap was a leading brand of soap in the market (it had nearly a twenty share of market). It was marketed as the soap that both cleaned and softened. It seemed a natural at the time to explore other areas where the two potential benefits of clean and soft would also fit. Extensive research was done, and it was interpreted literally—the dishwashing category was prime for a product positioning that purported "strong clean" (able to cut through grease and grime) and yet leave the hands feeling "soft and smooth." The introduction of "Madge," the nail care lady dipping her customers fingers in dishwashing liquid, was proof positive that this product was gentle to the skin. The "good news" was that Palmolive became one of the leading brands in dishwashing detergent; the "bad news" was that Palmolive Bar Soap's sales and share of market plummeted. Consumers couldn't wrap their minds around being able to "clean their face" and "do their dishes" with the same family of products. The result is that today Palmolive Bar Soap has less than a two share.[3]

In trying to understand the characteristics that make for successful mega-branding strategies, it appears that there are five principle components that apply:

- **A core brand must be the market leader in a category or niche segment.** Unilever's Vaseline Brand typifies this mega-branding principle. Vaseline Petroleum Jelly owned the petroleum jelly market (and still does) when it launched Vaseline Intensive Care Lotion in 1971. Within two years after its launch, Vaseline Intensive Care Lotion became the leading brand of hand lotion and still is the dominant player in the hand and body lotions.
- **It must have unique, meaningful benefits that are associated with it.** Again in the case of Vaseline, it already had the reputation of being a "great moisturizer." It had built-in trust ("if I use it on my baby, it also must be gentle for me"). Later, Vaseline Intensive Care Lotion built its reputation on being able to "absorb quickly into the skin" while not leaving the skin "feeling greasy." This is a great credit to Unilever's marketing and research and development departments, which were able to differentiate the Intensive Care sub-brand from the parent Vaseline in terms of "not being greasy" but still be a great moisturizer like Vaseline.
- **There must be a dogged commitment to maintaining the parent brand's equity long-term.** This means deciding what the brand is going to stand for, and more importantly, what it will not be! I believe the essence of this statement is captured extremely well by Raulee Marcus, who was the vice president

of marketing for Neutrogena. She says, "My primary focus was to protect the 'purity' of the Neutrogena franchise. Neutrogena stands for 'clean' and 'pure'. Any category which could not extend these benefits to all other Neutrogena segments were dismissed out of hand. Therefore, categories like deodorants or makeup (which cover up stuff) were not areas of interest."

- **There must be a continual investment in both marketing support and R&D.** Unilever was successful in building the Intensive Care brand name and providing it with its own set of unique properties because the company poured money into continued marketing support and its R&D effort. Vaseline Intensive Care Lotion has been the leading advertised brand in the hand lotion market for more than twenty years. Its spending level has consistently been maintained at approximately eight percent of sales. All the major mega-brands are supported in this manner—Neutrogena, Nivea, Colgate and Crest Dental Products, L'Oreal Hair Care Products, Helene Curtis' hair care products.
- **Last, but certainly not least, marketers must continually invest in consumer research to make sure that messages remain relevant to the core user group.** The objective is to ensure that no dissonance is set up between the parent brand and the line extensions.

A Case Study In Mega Branding
PROCTER & GAMBLE'S COSMETIC STRATEGY

In September 1995, Procter & Gamble started testing the Oil of Olay brand of color cosmetics in Evansville, Indiana food stores, drug stores, and mass merchandisers. This is a huge line that includes 114 items across lipstick, nail polish, eye shadow, blush, foundation formulas, and mascaras.[4]

With the emergence of Oil of Olay, Procter & Gamble will have three different cosmetic lines: Cover Girl, Max Factor, and Oil of Olay. Managing these lines successfully will depend on developing a perceived price/value relationship between each brand. In many ways, Procter & Gamble's Olay strategy is reminiscent of the Sears product line strategy of "good," "better," and "best." Procter & Gamble is banking heavily on getting this price/value relationship right.

Procter & Gamble executives view their three cosmetic lines in the following manner: "Oil of Olay's imagery will be more sophisticated than Cover Girl's clean fresh look; it will be aimed at Oil of Olay's core group of women 25 plus who have average to above average household incomes. However, it will not be positioned as a high glamour brand like Max Factor."[5]

Below is a depiction of the price/value dimension that Procter & Gamble is using in developing its cosmetic strategy:

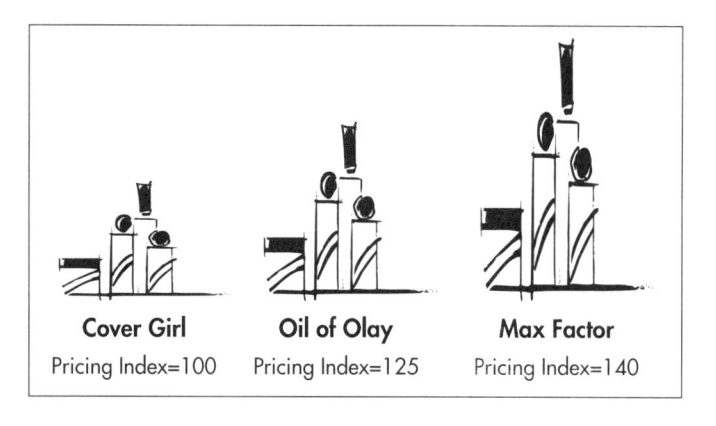

Cover Girl	Oil of Olay	Max Factor
Pricing Index=100	Pricing Index=125	Pricing Index=140

TALKING THE LANGUAGE OF "BEAUTY SCIENCE"

To get into most beauty care categories today, a "scientific" platform is still most helpful (the exceptions are fragrances, which is still driven by sensual imagery and some niche segments in hair care and skin care which play off a natural connotation). Images connoting the "wonders of biotechnology" for cosmetics, skin care, and hair care help the consumer equate product delivery with "performance." Current beauty care sub-segments abound with examples of high tech platforms—long lasting lipsticks, liposomes in facial products, AHA ingredients to help retard the aging process. Look for high tech improvements to not only continue, but to accelerate.

During the early to mid-80s, products and positionings using a "bio-tech" orientation were virtually the exclusive domain of the "prestige" brands (those sold only in department stores). However, since the introduction of L'Oreal's Plenitude in late 1989, these "high-tech" platforms have become as commonplace in the mass market as they are in department stores. Product descriptions that relate to "scientific" positionings that continue to garner significant interest among consumers include:

- Anti-Aging/Anti-Wrinkling
- Cellular Restoration
- Liposomes
- Replenishing, Rejuvenating, or Treating
- Anti-Drying
- Sensory Cues: Feel It/See It Working
- Recovery Complex/Turnaround Cream
- Self-Sealing
- Hair Volumizer
- Vitamin-Based Formulation
- Color Corrective
- Hypoallergenic/Fragrance Free
- Cover Cream Concealer
- Essential Moisturizers
- Nourishes Skin
- Dermatologist Tested
- Oil Free

Clearly, **marketers will continue to emphasize therapeutic positionings for skin care, cosmetics, and hair care.** Therefore, in developing targeted propositions, it seems that a beauty promise must be teamed with a "scientific reason why." The following partnerships appear to be working now and should continue to work in the future:

PROMISE	BENEFIT "THE WHAT"	INGREDIENT "THE HOW"
Skin/Cosmetics		
Makes Skin Younger Looking	Reduces Signs of Aging	Contains a Sunscreen
Makes Skin Feel Healthy	Moisturizes Skin	Replenishes Skin's Moisture Balance
Makes Skin Feel Firm	Makes Skin Stronger	Restores Damaged Skin
Makes Skin Soft & Smooth	Treats Dry & Cracked Skin	Penetrates Deeply Into The Layers Of The Skin
Fastest Drying Color	Dries In Minutes	Won't Smudge or Smear
Hair Care		
Fuller Hair	Add Volume	Extra Body Formula
Healthy/Shiny Hair	The More It's Used The Shinier Hair Gets; Bold Brilliant Color	Vitamin-Based Formula or Luminescent Gel
Fragrances		
Innocence; Passion; Mystery; Romance	Alluring Visual Image	Scent Differentiation

(Column group header: THE SCIENTIFIC REASON WHY)

ADEQUATE ADVERTISING AND SUPPORT LEVELS

Successful beauty care marketers have extraordinarily strong brand names with dominant market shares that are well supported with marketing dollars in terms of both advertising and trade and consumer promotion.

A number of years ago, Ogilvy and Mather did an exhaustive study of more than three hundred branded products. The study assessed brand profitability under strategies that were either advertising driven or promotion driven. The results showed that advertising dominant brands (where advertising accounted for an average of sixty-six percent of the marketing funds) had the highest return on investment (average thirty-one percent ROI versus eighteen percent ROI for brands that were dominant on the promotion front). **The Ogilvy study also revealed that changes in spending levels for media advertising positively related to share changes, while changes in spending for sales promotion did not significantly relate to market share change.**[6]

Beauty care brands spend on the average at least eight percent of their sales dollars in media on an annual basis. This appears to be one of the "price of entry characteristics" required to remain a major factor in the beauty care market.

CATEGORY COMMITMENT: UNDERSTANDING THE CONSUMER AND CONSISTENTLY IMPROVING THE PRODUCT PROPOSITION

Successful companies are committed to the categories that they are in; they're committed to finding a "better" way to do whatever they do. It means developing value-added products that have a meaningful difference and, more importantly, fulfill consumers' "need gaps." There is no doubt that consumers perceive value, and that there is a strong relationship between value and price.

Mike Perry, the former worldwide coordinator of personal care for Unilever, said it best when discussing why Unilever has had such success over the years: "Unilever understands the consumer better than any company in the world. Unilever studies, serves, respects, listens, fears, admires, knows the consumer, and recognizes the consumer as the center of the Unilever universe. Because of this consumer understanding, Unilever is able to provide strong concepts that explicate the consumer's needs. All divisions in Unilever see their business as selling concepts and using products as delivery forms."[7]

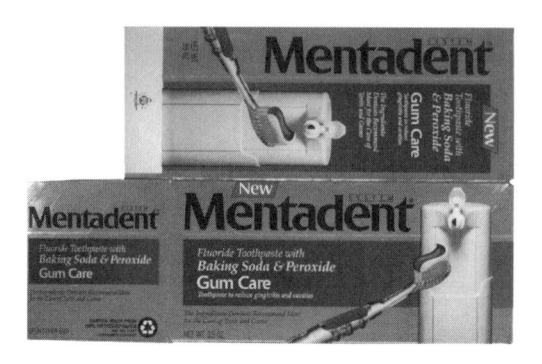

A Case Study
UNILEVER'S MENTADENT TOOTHPASTE

Mentadent Toothpaste is not strictly a beauty product (although white teeth certainly connotes beauty); however, its story typifies how successful products can be introduced through understanding generational marketing, marrying that knowledge with technological advances, developing a compelling advertising positioning, and then supporting it with marketing dollars.

Unilever's goal was to become the first company in the United States to successfully market a toothpaste that combined the "dentist recommended" benefits of baking soda and peroxide in a stable environment. The entry was introduced nationally in 1992, but it was a "work in progress" beginning in 1986.

Unilever knew that as the population ages, the concern for "gum health" would continue to soar. It also knew that the primary ingredients recommended by dentists to counteract "gum disease" were baking soda and peroxide. Yet baking soda and peroxide were not compatible ingredients. Each had to be encapsed in separate dispenser systems. This forced Unilever to create a package that was extremely different from current toothpaste products. The package involved a pump which held the two ingredients in separate tubes. This new pump was not only "bigger" than traditional pump offerings, but it also took up more shelf space and caused the product to be significantly more expensive than other toothpaste products (like tartar *control)*. Unilever turned each of these problems into a major consumer benefit through its marketing efforts:

- The pump became a "convenience" benefit.
- The higher price point made it "premium/special."
- The packaging gave it a unique shelf presence in the store.

Unilever put as much work into the positioning of Mentadent as in the formulation and packaging. Unilever also did not expect the brand to begin to payoff until it had been well-established in the marketplace. This gave the brand latitude to build a consumer base through extensive advertising and, more importantly, sampling. Today Mentadent is the third largest selling toothpaste brand at retail (behind Crest and Colgate).[8]

ADVERTISING STRATEGY: THE BIG IDEA

George Lois, one of the truly great visionaries of the modern advertising profession, stated in his 1991 book, *What's The Big Idea*, that **"The Big Idea will always be what great advertising is all about. If you can't describe the Big Idea in one sentence or in three or four words, you don't have a Big Idea."**

Lois goes on to define a Big Idea as: "a surprising solution to a marketing problem, expressed in memorable verbal and/or graphic imagery—it is the authentic source of communicative power."

Finding this elusive Big Idea is the first and most important dynamic in marketing. Without this, there is *no* marketing process. Lois presents a terrific visual in his book concerning a statement he attributes to Michaelangelo: "A sculpture is imprisoned in a block of marble, and only a great sculptor can set it free." This is also the essence of great advertising. Your Big Idea must be expressed in the language of the target consumer— she must be able to "see it," "feel it," and, most importantly, "want it."

The way to ensure that "great advertising" captures the Big Idea is through rigorous attention to copy strategy. Unilever, Colgate, L'Oreal, Revlon, and Calvin Klein have developed detailed means for integrating a brand's marketing strategy into its advertising copy (inclusive of point of sale information) because of the attention they give to the copy strategy document. The primary objective of the copy strategy is to provide clear, consistent direction to the creative group. It ensures that each separate piece of a brand's total advertising communication contributes towards building the desired consumer perception of the product (this assumes the agency has already been indoctrinated in the brand's key benefits and USP or unique selling proposition).[9] To guarantee that the copy strategy incorporates all the elements of the marketing strategy, it must address the following dimensions:

- **What is the competitive environment?** What products are you competing with? Where will you source your business?
- **Who are the target audience?** Who are you talking to?
- **What is the desired impression that you want to create for your brand?** This is frequently based upon the most leveragable "promise."
- **What should be the tone and manner or the brand personality?**

Calvin Klein has been tremendously successful over the past two decades. His advertising, although controversial, has been targeted specifically to has audience—Xers—for more than twenty years.

Who would have thought it possible that an identical fragrance could be marketed to both men and women?

A Case Study
CALVIN KLEIN'S CK ONE

CK one's success was based on the fact that the Klein organization is dedicated to understanding the mindset of Generation X users. They learned that the attitudes of Generation X men and women were similar in terms of their views of the future and their belief that they have a common goal: "to get to where the Boomers are today." The fact that Generation X men would prefer to work for a woman ("they are more understanding"[10]) speaks volumes as to why CK one was successful.

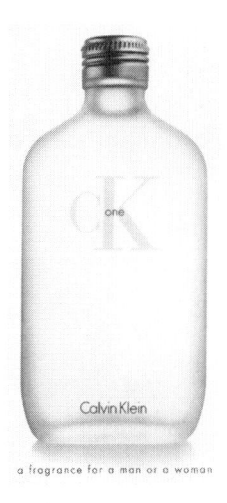

a fragrance for a man or a woman

Calvin Klein and CK one illustrate one of the main points of this book: **Most beauty care successes are well planned out and rooted in consumer lifestyle dynamics. They are based on marketers clearly understanding lifestyle trends and translating those ideas into tangible assets.** In a 1994 interview with Elle magazine, Calvin Klein described his process: "I start with a concept; really, it's an idea. It's based on maybe what's going on in society. We do market studies and have very sophisticated people analyzing what's going on, and then we all meet and we talk about it. When an idea comes out of that process, somehow it always relates to me. So it does get to be very personal. When the idea is fleshed out, I try to create an image of what the product is. Who am I attracting? Who do I think will wear this? Who will understand it? Lastly, the photograph (picture of the ad) has to say something to me that's emotional. It has to make my heart start beating. It has to do more than just convey the message of what the product is—it has to grab you. I want people to stop when they're turning the pages of the magazine. I want them to stop at our page and notice it."[11]

Calvin Klein is at the apex of the marketing process because he has continued to remain relevant to his target audience. The 1995 CK one fragrance launch was as successful as his 1980 Calvin Klein jeans program with its famous "nothing gets between me and my Calvins" tag line. Kate Moss (the current Klein spokesperson) and her grunge waif look has had as much impact as Brooke Shields' playful sensuality fifteen years earlier in the Calvin Klein jeans ads.

REFRESHING AND REINVENTING CORE FRANCHISES

All successful beauty care companies continually refresh and reinvent their core franchises. Importantly, they do it with meaningful product differentiation. One of the things that you will continue to see less of in the future are "me too" products (even in "new improved" formulations). Marketers finally have begun to understand that "me too" products only get you into a price game (price becomes the only leverageable variable). **If price becomes the primary inducement to buy, it will only lead to lower manufacturing margins—and ultimately less money for marketing. This is a losing business proposition.** Successful brands have stayed away from the price game by value-adding to their products—continually making them relevant to their core users. For example:

- Revlon improved its ColorStay Lipstick by value-adding a "long-lasting" additive. Long-lasting has since become a "price of entry" for all manufacturers across a myriad of cosmetic categories (eye care, makeup, and nail care to name a few).
- Procter & Gamble's addition of a conditioning agent to Pert shampoo virtually created a new category. 2-in-1 shampoo/conditioning products have become a mainstream segment in the $5 billion hair care market.
- Unilever's addition of an anti-aging ingredient to Pond's face care products has revolutionized a once staid product. To paraphrase, "it's not your mother's cold cream." It has become as vital a brand for the year 2000 as it was in the 1930s.

R&D investment has enabled these successful marketers to put forth meaningful line extensions and improved base brand formulations. Successful companies will continue to increase their R&D expenditures in their core categories in the years ahead.

It is imperative, however, to understand that there are different strategies and accompanying expenditures based on whether a company is "refreshing" a brand or "reinventing" a brand.[12]

REFRESHING A BRAND

This generally relies more on a conceptual (rather than a technical) point of difference. Innovation in packaging and/or form are contemporary "face lifts" that help brands to refresh their franchises. For example, both Ponds Cold Cream and Vaseline Petroleum Jelly refreshed their brand by going from a glass to a plastic container.

In cases like this, the primary marketing emphasis is at retail with point of sale merchandising (versus extensive on-air advertising expenditures). It should also require no new manufacturing expenses; only existing manufacturing facilities or capabilities should be used. Thus, "refreshment" should not add significant costs to the brand. In the case of both Ponds and Vaseline, these improvements were not only embraced by the consumer, but they also had the added internal benefit of lowering shipping and handling costs for Unilever (less chance of breakage and lighter case weights due to plastic).

Unilever wisely plowed back the savings from these package changes into marketing the brands via the "new news." Only after the story was told for both brands (and every potential user had "heard" the news) were the savings reflected in bottom line profit.

REINVENTING A BRAND

Reinventing a brand requires a technical and conceptual product breakthrough. To illustrate, a technical breakthrough requires a genuine product improvement—the addition of a "longer lasting" ingredient as in the case of Revlon's ColorStay Lipstick. A conceptual breakthrough is the promise of "looking different" at an individual's whim. This is at the root of success of temporary hair coloring products. The promise of instantly looking different is a huge incentive that is met by the equally alluring peace of mind that it doesn't have to be permanent if the person doesn't like the results.

It goes without saying that "reinventing a brand" requires a continued commitment to R&D (if only to ward off the competition) and it implies that there will be a long-term commitment to the brand from a corporate standpoint (particularly in terms of media support).

In the late 1980s and early 1990s, Revlon virtually abandoned the department store business and went after the mass cosmetic market. It reinvented the Revlon brand not only by redefining where its customer shops, but also by significantly refining its target market. Revlon's marketing focus had a clear generational skew— it exclusively went after the aging baby-boomers. Further, it also brought in a new management team that was schooled in marketing products to this segment. Kathy Dwyer, the senior marketing executive for Revlon, was formally from Clairol (Clairol's emphasis on its hair coloring business is squarely aimed at the Boomers). Dwyer's direction was "to deliver products to women that have both value and substance."[13] This was accomplished via the team approach. Under Dwyer's direction, marketing, R&D, and the advertising agency went to work to give women what they wanted: "less hype and better products."[14]

The first major result of this effort was the midsummer 1994 launch of ColorStay Lipstick.

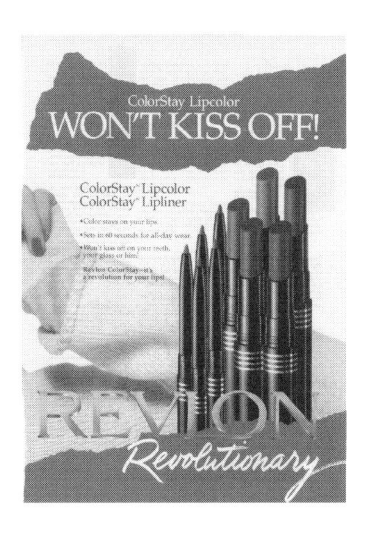

A Case Study
COLORSTAY LIPSTICK
The promise that this product won't "kiss off" or "rub off" and lasts for eight hours made it an instant success. To further support the added-value of this product, Revlon decided to launch this product at comparable prices to competition (as well as Revlon's own current lipstick products). This improvement in the value equation (significantly better product at a reasonable price) was critical in driving the growth of ColorStay.

Revlon had actually developed the ColorStay formula in the early '90s as part of their Ultima 3 department store line. However, rather than driving home the "long lasting" benefit, the management team at the time positioned the product as a new "sexy" formulation. Additionally, the target group was not clearly defined. Although the positioning under Ultima 3 was "young" in nature, the Revlon brand has an older Boomer skew. Thus, this was a huge disconnect in the marketing plan. As a result the Ultima 3 product went nowhere. Dwyer's repositioning of the product benefit (from "sexy" to "long lasting") coupled with a change in channel dynamics ("class to mass") and a clearly focussed target market (Xers to Boomers) made ColorStay a tremendous success. It also demonstrated the importance of companies understanding the R&D aspects of their businesses and appropriately marrying them to their consumer base.

The lesson in understanding Revlon's success is that a company can improve its bottom line while also improving products and holding back unnecessary price increases. The "reinventing" of Revlon was based squarely on understanding its core consumer. **The key was to ensure that product introductions solved major category problems. In the case of ColorStay, it was directed at the number one category need or gap: a long-lasting formula.**

THE MARKETING ELEMENTS NEEDED TO ENSURE COMPETITIVENESS

UNDERSTANDING MARKET DYNAMICS

You must understand market size and growth prospects, segmentation importance (the target segment you are aiming for), and the retail environment (with specific emphasis on trade channels).

UNDERSTANDING TRIAL/PURCHASING DYNAMICS

You also must understand usage incidence (the percentage of consumers that are using your category and product currently or are planning to use your product and category in the future), the purchase cycle and repeat rate, and brand awareness and distribution.

Understanding the market dynamics and trial/purchasing elements are fully explained and integrated in chapters 10–13.

UNDERSTANDING FINANCIAL DYNAMICS

TRADE ALLOWANCES

The most important dimension to plan for is the IGP (Initial Gross Profit) level. IGP is the amount of money available after the cost of goods has been subtracted from sales. Once this percentage is fixed, it sets the amount that a brand will have for marketing support. Manufacturers must walk a fine line between "need" and "greed" in establishing this level.

In the world of beauty care, my experience indicates that for the prestige class of trade (predominately the department store business), the margin requirements must ensure that a brand (regardless of beauty care category) has a minimum of a five percent advertising-to-sales ratio and at least a ten percent trade allowance level. However, beauty care products sold in the "mass" class of trade (food outlets, drug outlets, or discount stores) usually require a minimum advertising-to-sales ratio of eight percent and a trade allowance level of fifteen percent of sales (which often escalates to twenty percent or higher during the peak promotional seasons—Christmas, Mother's Day, Easter, etc.).[16]

ADVERTISING LEVELS

Beyond the absolute expenditure for advertising and promotion, it is important to understand the relative proportion of advertising spending and its impact on brand performance (and ultimately its profit contribution). By comparing a brand's share of market with its share of voice (its share of total advertising dollars spent in a specific category), marketers can ball-park the health of their franchise.

In 1990, James Shroer, a vice president of Booze, Allen & Hamilton, wrote a paper in the *Harvard Business Review* entitled, "Ad Spending: Growing Market Share." His research noted three different types of spending strategies:

- **Market leaders can have a share of voice somewhat less than their share of market.** A seventy-five percent share of voice to share of market ratio is acceptable because "leaders enjoy a scale advantage enabling them to outspend the followers at a lower per unit cost."[17]
- **Niche-oriented brands should maintain share of voice levels about equal to their share of market positions.** It's interesting that Shroer comes to this conclusion, since many smaller brands (under a five share of market) tend to significantly overspend by maintaining a share of voice that is much higher than their share of market.[18] His point is that this results in lower than necessary profits: "A smaller player cannot hope to win the spending war. In order to maintain profitability, a smaller competitor trying to exploit a differentiated niche should not try to grow beyond narrow limits because it would be folly to launch an ad offensive on the leaders."[19]
- To maintain his presence, the **midsize player (for example, the Number Two brand in a category) generally is forced to outspend Number One in terms of the relative relationship between a brand's share of market and its share of voice.**

Company Number Two is likely to be less profitable than Company Number One because the latter can maintain a competitive voice level while spending less than its "fair share." This talks to the difficulty of brands caught in the middle—between number one and smaller "niche" brands. Thus, without a well-defined consumer target, optimum profitability can't hope to be realized.

CLASS OF TRADE/PRICING CONSIDERATIONS

The IGP level will be influenced significantly by the type of "selling" arrangement the retailer has. Therefore, it is necessary to develop retail margin requirements based on an understanding of trade class influence.

FOOD-DRUG-MASS CLASS OF TRADE

EDLP (Everyday Low Price). This type of pricing policy is based on a certain percentage off "everyday" on a brand's suggested retail price. Procter & Gamble pioneered the EDLP concept in the early 1990s as a means for retailers to stop the escalation of increasing deal promotion levels (Wal-Mart was the first major retailer to implement the Procter & Gamble concept). As the 1990s close, however, the adage "be careful what you wish for" appears to be unfolding. **Thus, EDLP has begun to show a few "hiccups" in terms of consumer acceptance.** Since few beauty care products have their SRP (suggested retail price) on the package in the mass class of trade, consumers are skeptical that they are "getting a good deal."

EDLP in its purest form means that the price of a product is the same day in and day out. **Studies have indicated that consumers regularly shopping in an EDLP environment forget over time that the product is already priced at the lowest level.** Their perception after about a year is that the retailer is never giving them a break because the consumer never sees a lower price. The consumer tends to forget that the retailer already has the lowest price in the marketplace because she rarely shops around. This is particularly true for products bought in food stores (consumers tend to shop most often in only one food store).

In 1996, I did some work for Winn Dixie, a major grocery chain in the Southeast who adopted an EDLP strategy in 1994. When Winn Dixie consumers were asked about the prices at Winn Dixie, they said that they were higher or the same as their competitors. They complained that there were not enough sales or promotions. Nevertheless, Winn Dixie's consumers were much aware of the grocer's EDLP policy. **The lesson to learn: If a consumer never sees a price change, then she thinks she's not getting "a deal."**

EDLP works well on products that have an SRP stamped on their package, such as greeting cards. Why? Because then the consumer can always look on the back of a greeting card and determine if it is a real sale (SRP is always printed on the back of every greeting card).

High-Low Pricing Policy. Most retailers are still selling products based on the traditional high-low pricing strategy. Here, consumers pay a higher price than EDLP most of the time (approximately sixty percent of the year) while the remaining times they are buying "on deal." The deal component generally ranges between twenty and fifty percent,[21] with the exception of the ever-popular "Buy-1-Get-1-Free." Although this tends to be more expensive for the manufacturer than an EDLP policy, the consumer likes this type of price policy better. At least at some point in the year, the consumer truly believes she is getting a good deal. In her terms, she thinks that "I've beaten the system this time." This concept of "winning" is a key driver of the beauty care consumer's shopping value system.

EDLP as a policy will decline in the future; while Hi-Lo will be gaining. In a comprehensive study in 1994, University of Chicago researchers concluded (based on extensive testing with retailers in the Chicago market) that a Hi-Lo pricing policy not only makes consumers feel as if they are winning, but also it significantly enhances retailer profits.[22]

Since greed will continue to be a principal driver for retailers, they will be demanding more deals for their consumers. Manufacturers currently having an EDLP policy will not be able to afford these "incremental" promotions and maintain EDLP as their primary way of doing business.

DEPARTMENT STORE TRADE CLASS

The department store trade class has been changing the way it sells products. It is increasingly adopting some of the more successful tactics observed in the mass merchandiser trade class. More deals are being offered in the department store than at any other time in the past twenty years.[23] This is being driven by intense competition at retail (from alternative shopping formats such as supercenters, warehouse clubs, factory outlets, and direct mail as well as from the concentration that has occurred in the department store class of trade).

The fact that department stores are running more deals means that margins are beginning to erode across many prestige beauty categories. On top of this, gifts with purchase for skin care and fragrances have escalated in terms of offerings; this too has added to the eroding margin base. (It used to be only at Christmas; now it's year round.) Thus, the value consciousness of the consumer and her seemingly never-ending search for "the best price/value" will continue to put pressure on prestige manufacturers and retailers over the coming years.

Also exerting pressure on beauty care products in the prestige class is the concept that "fashion has become unfashionable."[24] This is being driven by the relaxation of dress codes in the workplace. In 1996, eighty percent of Fortune 1000 companies had at least one casual day, while thirty-five percent of these companies had full-time casual dress.[25] As "dress-up" becomes "dress-down," marketers will have to be extremely creative in this class of trade if they are to maintain their business.

One of the most telling figures in recent years that demonstrates the weakness inherent in the department store trade class is the fact it now accounts for only about twenty-five percent of apparel sales.[26] Clothing was once the bastion of the department store, but today's consumers think department stores are either "too expensive" or they are determined "to wait for a season ending great deal."

Nevertheless, certain beauty care manufacturers have been extremely successful in developing department store businesses in recent years. No one has done this better than Estee Lauder. Estee Lauder is the premier marketer in the prestige sector because it understands the core elements of generational marketing and marries them with an appropriate price point. (Estee Lauder knows the price/value equation better than anyone else in this class of trade.)

A Case Study

ESTEE LAUDER'S ORIGINS

An example of Estee Lauder's understanding of the price/value equation is its Origins beauty care line. Origins was introduced in early 1990 under an environmental positioning theme. It was designed to meet consumers' "green expectations."[27] The Origins product concept began nearly seven years before it actually was introduced nationally. The research department at Estee Lauder in the early 1980s was investigating the importance of the "green movement" vis-à-vis cosmetics. The research showed that there were three levels of environmentally concerned consumers:[28]

- *"True Blue Greens" who are willing to pay more for environmentally sensitive products.*
- *"Green Backs" who give to environmental causes and look for environmentally sensitive products.*

- "The Sprouts" who have shown an interest in buying environmentally sensitive products.

By 1990, these three environmentally concerned groups accounted for nearly fifty percent of the population.[29] Thus, Estee Lauder concluded there was an opportunity to develop a cosmetic line with the following positioning: **Products for Women Seeking a Healthy Lifestyle and a More Harmonious Relationship with Nature.**

In a 1991 press release, Estee Lauder's Rebecca C. McGreevy described Origins: "Origins is the first major cosmetics company to bring naturals and aroma therapy into the mainstream. Origins' commitment is to the total well-being of the individual. The line is intended to show that we are environmentally responsible, although we recognize that 'being green' is not our sole purpose for being. Nevertheless, the fact that plant extracts are used instead of animal derivatives and that no unnecessary aerosols, petroleum, or alcohol is added demonstrates the line's dedication to the environmental movement."[30]

Origins was successful because it had a single-minded dedication to providing a total beauty environment that is based as much on a "state of mind" as it is on product delivery.[31]

All the products are environmentally safe, all contain natural ingredients, all were made without the need for animal testing, all come in "green" recyclable packaging, and there is **knowledgeable and "eco-friendly" sales personnel at each Origins counter.** All these elements make for a cohesive marketing presentation to the consumer. When coupled with the fact that the products do not cost any more than other cosmetics, it presented an excellent price/value for the consumer. (Early on Estee Lauder understood that the consumer will not pay a significant upcharge for an environmentally safe product, yet the consumer would prefer to buy an environmentally safe *product if it were available at the price she normally would pay for a beauty care product.)*

ESTABLISHING THE "RIGHT" RETAIL PRICE POINT IN FOOD, DRUG, AND MASS MERCHANDISER TRADE CLASSES

In my view, the establishment of the "right price" is the critical embodiment of the "price/value" relationship. In effect, it predetermines the class of trade component. Jim Mozingo, the former vice president of trade relations for Kayser-Roth (and, for twenty-seven years, director of trade relations for Unilever's Chesebrough-Ponds Division), has developed an interesting approach to establishing the retail price point. His concept is an "everyday fair price." To implement an "everyday fair price" requires an in-depth understanding of the consumer's shopping and purchasing attitudes by class of trade.

FOOD STORE CLASS OF TRADE

Consumers who buy their beauty care products in food stores are expecting to pay an upcharge versus a drug store or mass merchandiser. The reason for this is that they are willing to pay a certain percentage more for the convenience of being able to purchase their cosmetics, skin care, or hair care products at the same time as they are buying their groceries. This fact is clearly evidenced by Information Resources, Inc.'s database. In more than ninety percent of cases, beauty care brands sold in food, drug, and mass merchandisers have their highest prices in food stores.[32]

The objective is to assess how much that percentage is going to be versus the other trade classes. This relationship needs to be developed early in the product development process because it is a critical parameter in determining both margin and contribution levels.

DRUG STORE CLASS OF TRADE

The drug store class of trade, once the leader in developing optimal consumer pricing policies, has been the hardest hit trade class in the 1990s from the vantage point of changing consumer dynamics. This trade class (which still accounts for an estimated thirty to thirty-five percent of total beauty care dollars) has seen a decrease of about ten points in its share of the beauty care market since the late 1980s.[33]

A Case Study
THE CHANGING FORTUNES OF THE DRUG STORE TRADE CLASS

The drug class of trade is a classic example in American business retailing of what changing times and the failure to recognize changes can do to an industry.

Prior to the explosive growth of the category killers in the 1960s and 1970s (mass merchandisers, supercenters, food/drug combo stores, etc.), drug was The Destination *for shopping beauty care products. Women liked the local neighborhood aspect of the environment and believed that there was more knowledgeable help in this chain than other outlets (this was a carry-over from the days of the "all knowing pharmacist"). There was also a significantly wider selection of alternative products and brands stocked for each category than in supermarkets, and the prices were "much less" than in department stores. Lastly, but perhaps most importantly, they especially liked the "intimacy" of shopping this channel (aisles never appeared to be crowded).*

In the late 1970s and early 1980s there were a number of events that shook the foundation of the American environment and, in turn, forever changed the context of "shopping drug"— runaway inflation coupled with a recessionary environment, the mass exodus from cities to the suburbs in terms of both consumers and corporations, and a rethinking of the price/value relationship.

The latter was a bimodal movement. You had both the opulence of the 1980s—"brand defines who you are"—coupled with a "desire on the part of the consumer to win" (defined by finding the best price/value relationship). As an answer to the price/value relationship[34] and the need for consumers to win, the late 1970s and 1980s saw the emergence of a new type of drug store known as the deep discounter (PharMor, Drug Emporium, and F&M). These deep discounters started taking off in the early 1980s and, by the end of the decade, represented nearly a third of all drug store sales. They combined the best of both worlds from a consumer's perspective—they had the lowest prices everyday and also frequently offered deals on top of those prices. Thus, the consumer had the benefit of an "everyday low price" with significant discounts throughout the year.

The problem was that the deep discount drug chains began to run into financial problems with the concurrent disappearance of inflation in the early 1990s and the increasing dominance of the "value merchandisers" (a $100 billion Wal-Mart, a $34 billion Kmart, a $32 billion revitalized Sears, and the influx of warehouse clubs and factory outlets). By 1995 these chains accounted for less than half of what they had been (F&M went out of business; PharMor closed more than half its doors; and Drug Emporium closed approximately ten percent of its stores).

The reason for discussing this channel in such length is to make the point that many manufacturers continued to move their business (through the mid to late 1980s) to these deep discounters; even while knowing or at least suspecting that they were having or were projected to have significant financial problems. By moving to these drug store discounters, it required marketers to even further improve their cost structures or lower their margin requirements. In the case of beauty care products, for the most part, margins were lowered. Thus, those marketers that abandoned or cut back their support to the stronger and bigger chain drug stores during the 1980s (Walgreens, Osco, CVS, RiteAid, Revco, and Eckerd) have felt their wrath in the late 1990s.

As category management and shelf optimization have become the banner of the 1990s, many of the manufacturers who embraced the deep discounters have not been able to recover the lost volume because the remaining chains have been managing down the number of items they will carry. Therefore, these chains will not "take them back" to the degree that they previously were represented.

MASS MERCHANDISER TRADE CLASS

Establishing the "fair price" in the mass merchandiser class of trade is probably the most important decision that a beauty care marketer faces. Since the late 1980s the mass merchandiser trade class has approximately doubled its importance level in terms of beauty care sales. (In 1995, it accounted for approximately twenty-five percent of total beauty care sales.)[35] In discussing this trade class one need think of only three retailers (Wal-Mart, Kmart, and Target). Together they account for about eighty percent of total mass merchandiser sales (Wal-Mart, fifty percent; Kmart, twenty-five percent; and Target, ten percent).

The remaining twenty percent of mass merchandisers are comprised of regional retailers (Caldors, Bradleys, Ames, Hills). These retailers are either in, on the brink of, or have just come out of Chapter 11.

The most cogent way of developing the necessary data to establish a fair price point in mass merchandisers is to talk directly to each of these chains' consumers. As a class of trade, the loyalty level of these consumers are unparalleled. Nearly seventy percent of the consumers who shop for products in this channel would not even think of shopping anywhere else.[36] This is particularly true for Wal-Mart shoppers—they are the most satisfied shoppers across any retail channel or store.

Although each mass merchandiser has set specific margin requirements, there is some latitude to deal if you can demonstrate conclusively (through consumer research with their shoppers) that an item should sell for X rather than the retailer's desire for Y. I have seen each of these retailers back off their requirements (to a degree) in favor of their ultimate boss—their own shoppers.

CONCLUSIONS

Establishing brand saliency is the number one job of the marketer. This must be done through a combination of real and perceived product benefits and adequate dollars to establish consumer awareness for the brand. This can only be accomplished if a reasonable return on investment can be developed.

A critical element in developing the appropriate return on investment is the need to establish a "fair price" in the "right" class of trade. **The fair price concept ensures an adequate return to the manufacturer, such that the brand can be appropriately supported; the retailer will have enough of a return to continue to promote and sell the product; and the consumer will feel she is getting a "fair deal."** The embodiment of how successful a marketer can be is the brand's market share level (share takes into consideration marketplace dynamics, competitive forces, and a company's own marketing events).

From a consumer's standpoint, the price/value equation is composed of both functional and emotional components that go across a spectrum of consumer attitudes, wants, and needs. The next chapter discusses the primary beauty care market segments and the basic values inherent in each segment. Understanding how to manipulate these elements will dictate success or failure in marketing beauty products.

Chapter 4

OVERVIEW: THE WOMEN'S BEAUTY CARE MARKET

THE ART OF SUCCESSFULLY MARKETING to specific consumer segments is based on understanding three elements:

- Functional and emotional attitudes of each segment.
- Primary "hooks" to motivate each segment.
- Size and growth prospects of each segment.

In the late 1980s, *Glamour* and *Self* magazines both did beauty care segmentation studies. In 1994, Kayser-Roth (the second largest women's hosiery company in the world and maker of No nonsense, Calvin Klein, Hue, and Burlington legwear) updated its 1990 Legwear Segmentation analysis. In 1995, *Glamour* updated its 1988 study.[1] The segmentation discussed in this chapter is a blending of these studies and provides a definitive picture of the women's beauty care market. Each segment will be discussed in terms of its size; who comprises the segments from both an attitudinal, demographic, and socioeconomic standpoint; the products that they are most likely to use; and more importantly, where the segments will be in the year 2000.

A critical part of successfully marketing beauty care products is the need for marketers to have a future outlook (this is the reason that the segments are projected to the year 2000). All to often there is a tendency on the part of marketers not to go beyond what they know today. **For companies to be truly successful, they must take an "educated guess" about the future and not be afraid that it might be wrong.** The successful companies have done this across all product categories.

Ian Morrison in his 1996 book, *The Second Curve,* refers to forces that invariably will cause marketing organizations to have a future outlook or perish. Two of these, in particular, have significant implications for beauty care organizations:

- **Understanding the effects of new technologies.** "New technologies create the discontinuance of established businesses."[2] Examples abound in beauty care marketing—the introduction of anti-aging products in skin care, long-lasting formulations in cosmetics, the addition of conditioners in shampoo products, and the increasing use of micro-encapsulation technology in fragrances.
- **Understanding the new consumer.** Morrison defines this as "the anything, anytime, anyplace consumer".[3] He describes this new consumer as "smarter, richer, choosier, and more demanding. Today's consumers have high expectations in quality, service, design, and enough force to change the type of products and services coming to market and to transform the way products and services are sold."

Guessing about the future is particularly important for new products. It requires the marketer to pre-select a segment and develop a unique "reason why" for choosing that particular brand.

This "reason why" is based on a combination of both functional and emotional dimensions.

THE PRIMARY BEAUTY CARE SEGMENTS

As noted by Morrison, beauty care companies face the challenge of trying to build businesses in increasingly complex markets. Further, many of these categories (as well as segments within these categories) are mature businesses that already are proliferated with different brands, different formulations within brands (for example, scented to unscented products), and different SKUs (stock keeping units) within formulations (small sizes to large sizes within unscented and scented formulations). The key to success will be to identify the most profitable consumer segments that are underdeveloped to ensure maximum return on investment.

The four primary segments that comprise the women's beauty care market are the Fundamentalist, Traditionalist, Mature Stylist, and Impressionist. The chart on page 74 summarizes their differences.

Each of the four segments also comprise a combination of functional and emotional traits as well as feel and appearance characteristics.

- **Functional traits refer to delivering "price of entry" category benefits.** For example, facial moisturizers must deliver on the promise of "softer and smoother skin"; cosmetics must provide long-lasting color application; a hairspray has to "hold"; and a perfume must have a long-lasting scent.
- **Emotional traits provide the means for integrating a product's functional features into consumers' lives.** It is the essence of "why" a consumer chooses one brand over another. For example, L'Oreal's signature line, "I'm worth it," or Clairol's Ultress hair coloring statement, "Make Him Drop The Remote

WOMEN'S BEAUTY CARE MARKET SEGMENTATION

FUNDAMENTALIST	TRADITIONALIST	MATURE STYLIST	IMPRESSIONIST
Functionally based	Functionally based (but much less so than Fundamentalist)	Emotionally based	Emotionally based (almost to the extreme)
Inner directed	Inner directed (but "wants to fit in"/not be conspicuous)	Outwardly directed (are generally leaders and achievers)	Outwardly directed (defined by what she wears; must be center of attention)
Uninvolved	Buys mass brand names/Buys on sale	Involved shopper	Extremely involved shopper (believes in the promises of beauty care products)
Price shopper/Private label	Believes beauty products can help you look better	Brand names important/High loyalty to her brands	Looking good is more important than feeling good
Light user	Moderate user	Heavy user/Early adopter of new products	Experimenter (first to buy)
Buys in food stores/discounters	Buys in drug stores	Buys in department stores	Low brand loyalty/Low store loyalty
35+/Lower education/Income below $25M	40+/High School grad/Lower-middle income ($25-35M)	30-40 something/College educated/$40M+ household income	Under 35 years old/High school education/Medium to low household income ($20M-35M)

Control," are different yet equally motivating lifestyle positionings. (L'Oreal is inner directed; Clairol is clearly directed outwardly.)

- **Feel and appearance characteristics are specific product benefits that separate brands from one another.** Revlon's ColorStay Lipstick's appearance benefit is equated with "lasting"; Helene Curtis' Finesse Conditioner's feel dimensions are translated into a "variable conditioning" positioning. Finesse's slogan, "sometimes you need a little, sometimes you need a lot," is indicative of the technological product benefit. These are examples of brands carving out unique product niches.

The diagram on the following page characterizes the women's beauty care market along a two-dimensional axis.

SEGMENT GROWTH

The Fundamentalists and Mature Stylists groups will see the most growth through the remaining 1990s. The Fundamentalists have grown in direct response to the more casual lifestyles that typify the 1990s, while the Mature Stylists group has increased as a result of favorable aging dynamics. The size and change patterns of the four segments are shown below:

SEGMENT IMPORTANCE	1988	1994	1999
Segment I: The Fundamentalists	22%	25%	27%
Segment II: The Traditionalists	28%	26%	25%
Segment III: The Mature Stylists	24%	27%	29%
Segment IV: The Impressionists	26%	22%	19%

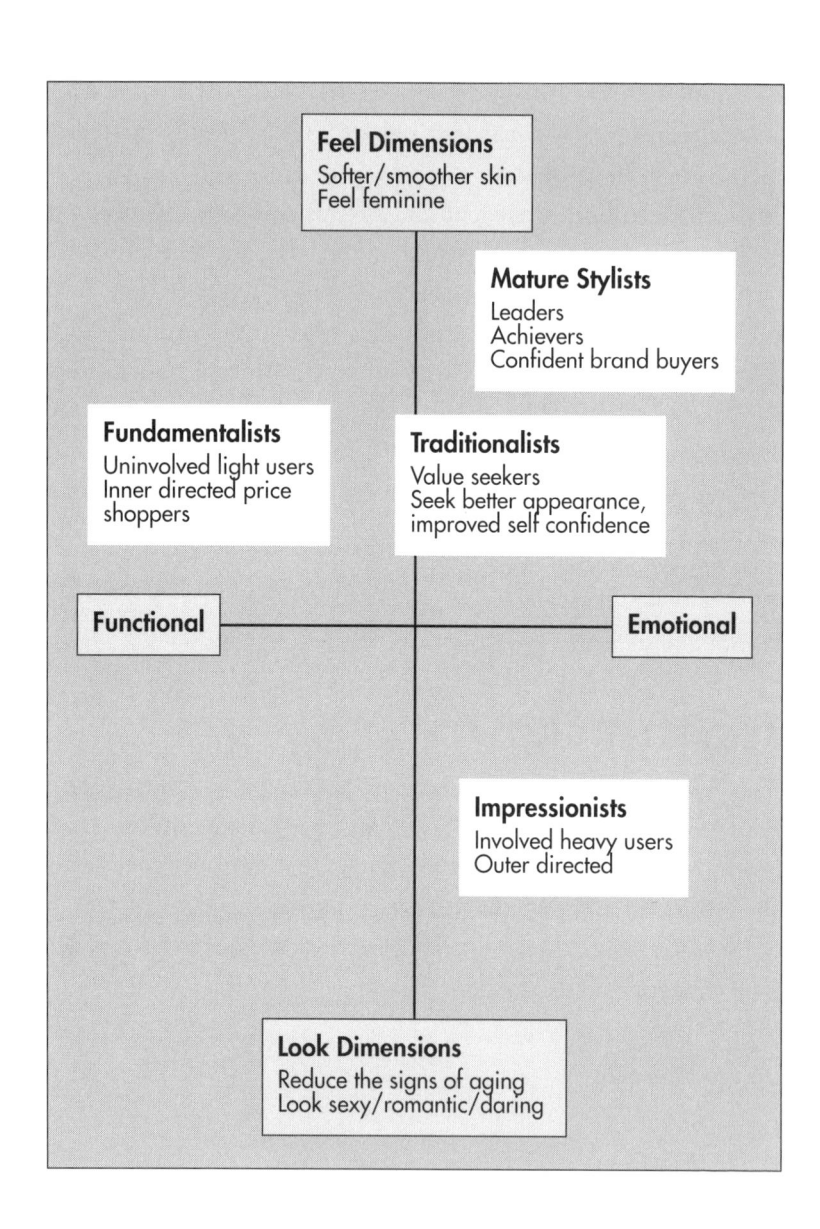

Feel Dimensions
Softer/smoother skin
Feel feminine

Mature Stylists
Leaders
Achievers
Confident brand buyers

Fundamentalists
Uninvolved light users
Inner directed price shoppers

Traditionalists
Value seekers
Seek better appearance, improved self confidence

Functional ——————————— **Emotional**

Impressionists
Involved heavy users
Outer directed

Look Dimensions
Reduce the signs of aging
Look sexy/romantic/daring

Chapter 5

WOMEN'S BEAUTY CARE SEGMENTATION

THE FUNDAMENTALIST

THE FUNDAMENTALIST TENDS TO BE an inner-directed individual who basically does not like to "bother" with beauty care products. Compared to the other three segments (Traditionalists, Mature Stylists, and Impressionists), she remains relatively uninvolved. Her primary goal is to use as few products as possible, and when she does use them, she is concerned with function over fashion. **She chooses beauty care products based on functional features (such as "easy to use" or "priced right") rather than fashion dimensions.**

Although she worries about ingredients damaging her skin (allergic reactions) and is concerned with the cost of beauty care products, she still has one overriding wish: to be more attractive. And so, she is willing to put up with the "necessary evils" of beauty care products. She also readily admits that she needs help in selecting beauty care products and in using and applying products (particularly cosmetics).

Demographically, she is "thirty-something" or older. She distinguishes herself by being "a low price shopper" and is slow to adopt new products. However, she also is concerned that her expenditure is "protected." Thus, a "money-back" satisfaction guarantee motivates the Fundamentalist to purchase. Because she does not believe that beauty care products "define her," she tends to purchase the majority of her products in either food stores (because of the convenience of buying it along with grocery items) or discount stores ("because they always have the cheapest price").

Since the Fundamentalists are least concerned with beauty and outward appearance, they are most open-minded about using "all family" or "unisex" products to satisfy their beauty care needs. Given their concern for economy, this type of positioning has great appeal.

The Fundamentalists' relatively low interest in beauty care products (particularly cosmetics) leads to low levels of brand loyalty. **Nevertheless, the concept of value, if positioned correctly, can be an important brand discriminator.** In this regard, products such as Maybelline's nail enamel can be quite appealing to Fundamentalists. "Quick drying/long lasting" nail enamel has appeal because it indicates "simplicity" as well as price/value.

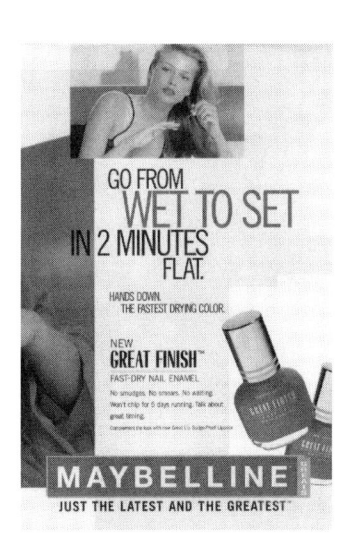

A Case Study

MAYBELLINE NAIL ENAMEL

In March 1996, Maybelline introduced its "Great Finish Fast-Dry Nail Enamel." Its headline—"Go from WET TO SET in 2 Minutes Flat"—is an ideal expression of what the Fundamentalist is looking for in cosmetics (function over fashion). The benefit of "quick drying" is an important value-added functional feature. When coupled with the "implied" guarantee of "No smudges. No smears. No waiting. Won't chip for 5 days running," it's a natural to get strong trial from this segment.

CONCLUSION: HOOKS FOR MARKETING TO THE FUNDAMENTALIST

➻ Market functional product features.
➻ Position products as "all family."
➻ Maintain low prices and frequent deals with money-back guarantees.

THE TRADITIONALIST

The Traditionalist is generally a self-conscious individual who has an aversion to attracting attention. The Traditionalist is in many ways the bridge between the Fundamentalist and the Impressionist and Mature Stylist. She is a "determined moderate" and "average" user of beauty care products. She has an inherent belief that beauty care products do "help her fit in" by making her as attractive as she can be. Inherently, she does not feel "dressed" without her beauty regimen.

From a marketer's vantage point, the Traditionalist is a relatively easy target. She is a believer in brand names and, generally, tends to stick with them. She is a "smart shopper" and prides herself in making the "best price/value" decision she can. Unlike the Fundamentalist, she is not the lowest price shopper (she generally would not buy a private label product), but she is concerned with getting the "best deal" on branded merchandise.

Traditionalists generally shop for their beauty care products in drug stores and discounters. They like the atmosphere of the drug store, which is less crowded than discounters or department stores (and, therefore, the Traditionalist feels less self-conscious buying products). Drug stores also offer a wide variety of products and have "expert advisers"—this dates back to the Traditionalist's belief in the pharmacist as a knowledgeable authority figure.

Traditionalists shop in discounters for the selection and, more importantly, price. Discounters reinforce their image of being a "smart shopper." Also, as discounters evolve, the new supercenters (primarily Wal-Mart, Kmart, and Target) have made their beauty care departments much more "destination shopping centers."

Traditionalists don't feel "dressed" unless they have their "outside face" on. **Traditionalists want to "fit in" as opposed to Mature Stylists and Impressionists, who "want to be noticed."** This is an important distinction in positioning products.

Overall, this group will be more receptive to a theme that stresses inwardly directed positionings ("want to feel better about myself") than more outwardly directed copy ("want to feel more attractive to others").

Demographically, the Traditionalists tend to skew older (40+), be family oriented, and come from middle to lower-middle income households (generally between $25,000 to $35,000).

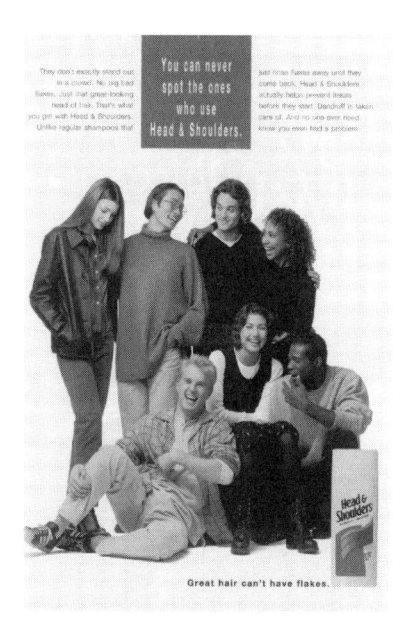

A Case Study
HEAD & SHOULDERS

The Head & Shoulders print execution talks effectively to Traditionalists. The slogan, "You Can Never Spot the Ones Who Use Head & Shoulders," is a compelling concept to this segment. Head & Shoulders is a premium priced product. However, this group will pay a premium for an over-the-counter product that helps them solve not only a physical problem (itchy scalp) but also an emotional concern (everyone notices you if you have dandruff). Hence, the Head & Shoulders promise of relief combined with "anonymity" is quite powerful. And so, even though it is a premium priced mass market shampoo, its value-added benefit makes the incremental cost a "fair" price to Traditionalists.

CONCLUSION: HOOKS FOR MARKETING TO THE TRADITIONALIST

- Use a problem/solution positioning orientation—aging, dry skin, thin hair.
- Market multifunctional products, such as products that clean and moisturize or leave skin smooth and soft.
- Emphasize price/value relationship—reinforce their belief in being a "smart shopper."

THE MATURE STYLIST

From a marketing viewpoint, the Mature Stylists is the most important group to beauty care marketers. Demographically, they are "thirty- to fortysomething" and are predominately working women with relatively high household incomes ($40,000+). They are not only the **largest segment** currently in the population, but they also are the **fastest growing group.**

Although they tend to be traditional in their views, the Mature Stylists are extremely fashion oriented. They want their beauty care products to reflect who they are—leaders and achievers. They revel in the fact that they "play" many roles: businesswoman, wife, and mother. They believe in brand names and, generally, will pay "big bucks" for their beauty care products. They make up the highest percentage of department store shoppers (nearly forty percent regularly buy their beauty care products in department stores)[1]; but they also are frequent purchasers of beauty care products in drug stores and discounters. Although this may sound like a contradiction, they are oriented toward being considered a "smart shopper" and, therefore, they do have a "value orientation." Value, however, does not mean the "lowest price" as in the case of the Fundamentalists. Rather, to the Mature Stylists, value means the best product at the best price. To a degree, they are willing to let the **brand name validate their purchase because it helps define who they are** (not surprisingly, they are the primary purchasers of designer labels).

Mature Stylists also tend to be early adopters of products. They believe in the "miracle of science," and so, they are the first to buy "technologically advanced" products. Anti-aging creams, cellulite reducers, chemical peels, liposuction, all are magical words to them. Their focus primarily is directed outwardly ("I want to look more attractive"). They use many products and, therefore, their total outlay for beauty care is much higher than either the Traditionalists or the Impressionists. (Impressionists tend to have lower incomes than Mature Stylists; they use knock-offs, private labels, or lower priced beauty products.)

Mature Stylists are **extremely brand loyal;** it is difficult to get them to try a new brand. More than anything else, the Mature Stylist (as well as the Impressionist) uses beauty care products to "feel feminine." Because of the many roles that they are asked to play, Mature Stylists think of beauty care products as being "an expression of personality and/or mood." **Additionally, they have an underlying belief that skin care products and cosmetic products are "good for the skin" because they help users "look their best."**

Mature Stylists are extremely heavy users of beauty care products primarily as a result of the tough stance they take toward the aging process. As a result, regimen products for skin care and cosmetics are important to this group. Mature Stylists have a deep, unabiding belief in the notion that "scientifically created skin care products" will significantly help reduce dryness, wrinkles, and in general, retard the aging process.

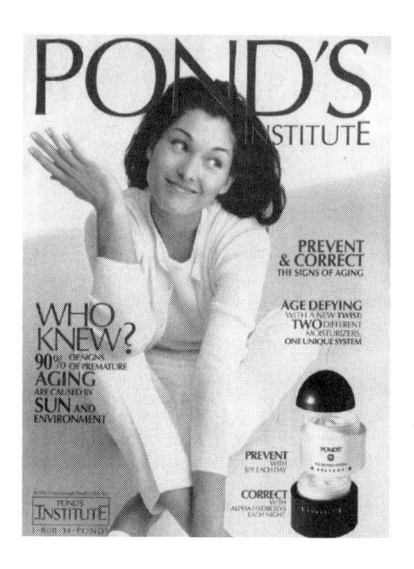

A Case Study
POND'S AGE DEFYING SYSTEM

Pond's Age Defying System is a terrific example of a product that plays to the Mature Stylist's concerns—aging and dry skin. It also provides a classic example of a problem/solution positioning approach. The Pond's print ad reads: "Who knew 90% of the signs of premature aging are caused by sun and environment?" Importantly, this product is put forward as a system (a regimen), which could be the norm for most beauty care products in the future. The payoff, however, is a potent promise—"Prevent & Correct the Signs of Aging." (It is probably the most powerful statement you can make to Mature Stylists.)

A particularly effective means for marketing new products to this key segment are through product samples. Forty percent of

Mature Stylists said that they bought their cosmetic products after they received a "free" sample.[2] Also effective, particularly because of the Mature Stylist's propensity to shop department stores, is to provide in-store demonstrations. In-store sampling provides a chance to try the product at no cost (obviously a real value hook) and to properly learn how to use the product (via the in-store demonstrator's expertise). In-store sampling also takes the "risk of use" out of the equation by allowing the individual to see the product "work" on others.

CONCLUSION: HOOKS FOR MARKETING TO THE MATURE STYLIST

➥ Marketing a brand name is a critical inducement to this segment.
➥ Positioning always must be outwardly directed and must reinforce the notion that Mature Stylists are leaders and achievers.
➥ Product introductions should convey a technological orientation such as anti-aging properties, aromatherapy sensory stimulation, or micro-encapsulation.

THE IMPRESSIONIST

The Impressionist is also a prime beauty care target. Her world is outwardly directed and, as such, she wants to "strut her stuff." She enjoys attracting attention and is disappointed if she is not the center of attention. If there is a new product on the market, you can be sure she was the first to try it.

The Impressionist tends to be younger (generally under 35), a working woman, but not necessarily an "upwardly mobile" individual. Impressionists are as likely to be secretaries and support staff as marketing and sales executives. Therefore, they are defined by what they wear, when they wear it, and how they wear it rather than "what they do."

The Impressionist has an unbridled belief that beauty care products are part of her wardrobe and that they are generally "good for the skin" and "good for the soul." To the Impressionist, looking good is as important (if not more important) than "feeling good." To a large extent, this segment is almost a throwback to another era in that the Impressionist seeks approval first from a man and then from her girlfriends. She believes in the power and promises of beauty care products—"they can (and do) make you better than you are." To this emotionally based group, "perception is everything."

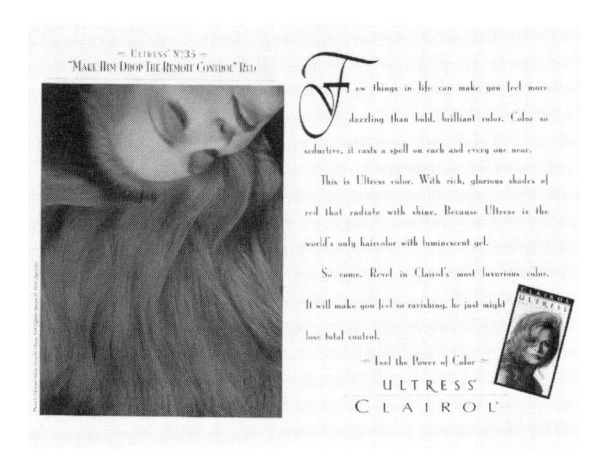

A Case Study

CLAIROL'S ULTRESS

Clairol's Ultress captures the Impressionist's feelings better than most hair care product print executions. From the ad's opening statement, "Few things in life can make you feel more dazzling," to its ultimate payoff, "it will make you feel so ravishing he just might lose total control," this ad zeros in on the Impressionist's key reason for being—getting her mate. In fact, the tag line, "Make Him Drop the Remote Control," could be a signature for all the Impressionist's beauty care product purchases.

Not surprisingly, the Impressionist uses more products than any other segment. When queried about their beauty care ritual (which is a vigorous one), Impressionists are the only group to say: "I want to feel sexy and be noticed." This aggressive, outwardly directed mindset is the "reason why" the Impressionist is sought after and fought over by every beauty care marketer.

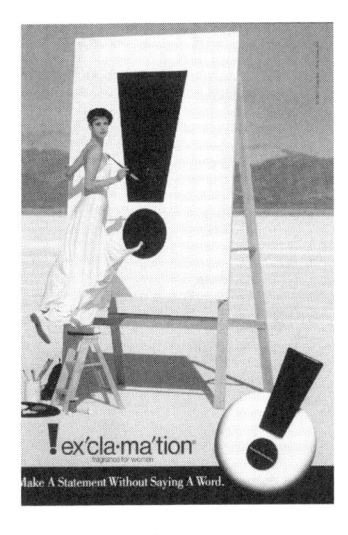

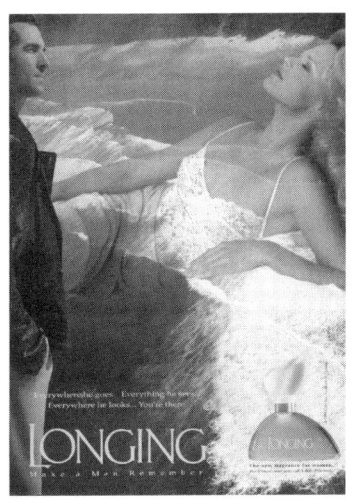

A Case Study
!EX'CLA-MA'TION AND LONGING
!ex'cla-ma'tion and Longing fragrances for women have just the right tonality for today's Impressionists. Together, the two have captured the most important dimensions of the Impressionist's needs: "attention getting" and "romance."

The !ex'cla-ma'tion headline reads: "Make a statement without saying a word." While Longing says: "Everywhere he goes… Everything he sees… Everywhere he looks … You're there."

Impressionists want to "impress others" and "feel sexy." These are the "reasons why" they are continually trying new brands. (Impressionists exhibit a lower than average loyalty index.)

Impressionists are an expensive segment to market to. They require sampling, in-store demonstrations, and regular "promotional sales" (inclusive of gifts with purchase in the department store trade class). This is the type of segment that would dump a brand for a designer knock-off (providing it worked).

This group, more than the Mature Stylists, is comprised of readers of magazines (nearly two-thirds regularly read fashion and beauty magazines to find out "what's new").[3]

Impressionists continually switch between products to create moods. For example, in hair care they alternate between mousses and gels—mousses to create volume and gel to create dramatic touches (like "the wet look").

This group was twenty-two percent of total women in 1994, but there has been a steady decline in their importance. By the year 2000, **further erosion will occur in the importance of this segment.** The reason is its demographic composition; because Impressionists generally are younger beauty care users (under 35), their numbers will be increasing far less over the next five years than the older population. Hence, the Mature Stylists, as a group, will be growing significantly faster because they will be riding the more favorable "Boomer age wave."

CONCLUSION: HOOKS FOR MARKETING TO THE IMPRESSIONIST

- Positioning must convey that a beauty care product will help them garner "approval from the man in their life" or even help get them one.
- Positioning also must convey the Impressionist's "outward nature" and need to be noticed. Conveying playful sexiness works well with this segment.

SEGMENTATION SUMMARY: THE HYPOTHETICAL MARKET BASKET

PRODUCT CATEGORY	FUNDAMENTALIST	TRADITIONALIST	MATURE STYLIST	IMPRESSIONIST
SHAMPOO & CONDITIONER	Suave	Finesse or Pert Plus	Vidal Sassoon	Pantene
HAIR COLORING	None	Nice 'N Easy	Preference by L'Oreal	Ultress
HAND & BODY LOTION	Jergens	Vaseline Intensive Care	Estee Lauder Resil Elastin Reform Cream	Almay
FACE CREAM	None	Pond's Age Defying System	Oil of Olay	Alpha Hydroxy Face Cream & Lotion
COSMETICS	Maybelline or Cover Girl	Max Factor or Revlon	Revlon, Estee Lauder or Elizabeth Arden	Clinique or Lancome
FRAGRANCES	None	Jontue or Charlie	Elizabeth Taylor's Passion or White Diamonds	Georgio or Primo (Knock-off of Georgio)

Women's Beauty Care Market Segmentation **89**

➻ The marketing program should be driven by print. Although print takes longer to "break through" to consumers than television executions, it is a more cost-effective means for reaching this target.
➻ To induce trial, sampling should be part of the program.

BEAUTY AND THE BEASTLY MARKET

PART II

TAMING UNCERTAINTIES IN ...

CHAPTER 6: MARKETING COSMETICS

CHAPTER 7: MARKETING HAIR CARE

CHAPTER 8: MARKETING SKIN CARE

CHAPTER 9: MARKETING FRAGRANCES

Introduction

THE BEAUTY CARE SUBSEGMENTS

TO SUCCESSFULLY MARKET BEAUTY CARE PRODUCTS, you must understand the fundamental category drivers behind each segment and develop motivating positionings for them. These "drivers" commonly referred to as "price of entry" category benefits are the primary reasons why consumers use specific categories:

DRIVERS

- A hand lotion must moisturize.
- A shampoo must clean.
- A nail polish must leave a "high shine."

Success or failure in beauty care marketing depends on differentiating between these price of entry characteristics in a **unique** way. For example, cosmetics is a color-driven business. Having a wide variety of colors to choose from is the price of entry. However, within each segment of cosmetics (lipstick, nail enamel, eye makeup, and face makeup), there also are basic consumer "wants" and "needs." Lipsticks must not only come in a wide color assortment, but they also should "last through the day." Thus, long lasting can become a primary positioning platform.

Positionings also can be developed based on an "absence of negatives." These commonly are referred to as secondary benefits. For example, all hand and body lotions must moisturize. However, some brands are "less greasy" than others. Therefore, a platform for a hand lotion based on "not being greasy" can have merit.

Although much marketing is based on an absence of negatives, positioning a product around the absence of a negative is not strong marketing. Since an absence of negatives (such as "not being greasy") is not the "reason why" an individual purchases a product, it generally does not garner the same consumer interest as a positioning based on a price of entry benefit (moisturizing, cleaning, protecting).

Chapters 6–9 detail the principal category positionings based on both primary and secondary drivers. Each section also includes examples of successful as well as unsuccessful positionings.

At the end of each chapter, there is a summary of the chief means for delivering a salient positioning. In reviewing these, it's important to notice that they have been divided into two components—primary drivers (price of entry benefits) and secondary drivers (the absence of negatives). Remember that although the high road is to develop positionings based on the primary drivers, many marketers have successfully "refreshed" their brands through the introduction of new improved formulations that were based on delivering secondary benefits.

Chapter 6

MARKETING COSMETICS

MARKET DYNAMICS

IN 1995, THE COSMETIC MARKET was an estimated $6.6 billion.[1] From 1987 through 1995, market growth for this industry was less than modest—about three percent per annum which was even below the four percent pace of inflation.[2] However, in mid-1994 and throughout 1995, the category heated up—in 1995, the total cosmetic category averaged a six percent dollar volume increase over 1994 levels.[3] This growth was primarily driven by the efforts of mass marketers Revlon, L'Oreal, Maybelline, and Procter & Gamble's Cover Girl. Each introduced new products with significant improvements in formulations and supported them with advertising, strong merchandising, and promotional presentations.

The cosmetic category is composed of four primary segments: facial makeup, eye makeup, lipstick, and nail enamel.

1995 COSMETIC MARKET SEGMENT IMPORTANCE

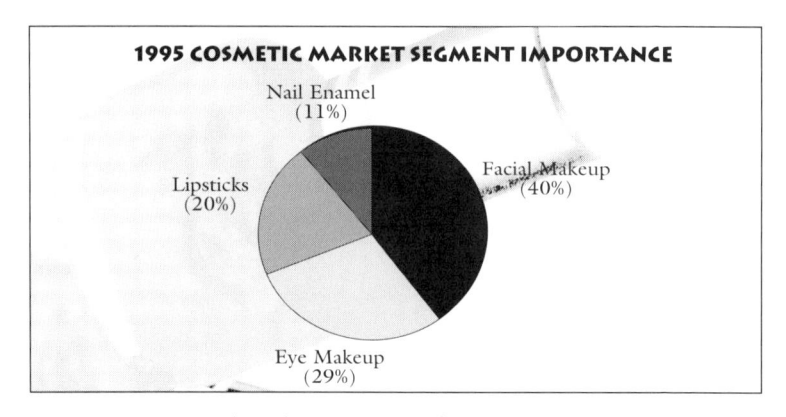

- Nail Enamel (11%)
- Facial Makeup (40%)
- Lipsticks (20%)
- Eye Makeup (29%)

Source: Cosmetic Market Volume Segments: Information Resources, Inc. (52 Weeks Ending 3/24/96); Total Cosmetic Market: Beauty Product Marketing (July/August 1988) Consumer Expenditure Study; "What's Driving Cosmetic Sales?" *Drug Store News*, Vol. 17, No. 9 (June 6, 1995); "Women On A Fast Track," *U.S. News and World Report*, Vol. 119, No. 18 (Nov. 6, 1995).

In viewing this industry, there is a significant distinction between "mass" marketers (those that sell cosmetic products in food stores, drug stores, and mass merchandisers) and "class" marketers (those that sell cosmetics in department stores). In 1995, department store cosmetic dollar volume sales was estimated at $4.3 billion while mass market cosmetics was $2.3 billion.[4] This relationship between mass and class has been relatively consistent throughout the past decade.

This ratio has been stable for so long because mass market companies traditionally have been "long on imitation and a bit short on innovation."[5] However, s**ince 1994, the mass market cosmetic manufacturers have been developing cutting-edge technologies and, as a result, they have grown faster during this period than prestige manufacturers.**

NAIL ENAMEL

The nail enamel segment represents only about seven percent of the total U.S. cosmetic market (approximately a $400 million business or roughly fifty-six percent of the total nail care sector),

96 *Beauty and the Beastly Market*

and yet, it was responsible for introducing color cosmetics to the market worldwide. This particular sector clearly defines what can happen when a company and/or person has a vision and the steadfastness to follow it. It is as much a story about vision as Steve Jobs with Apple or Bill Gates with Microsoft back in the early 1980s. The recap below is a distillation of the work done by Bud Brewster in the December 1995 edition of *Cosmetics and Toiletries*. His article was entitled, "50 Years of Cosmetic Color."

Case Study

THE REVLON STORY

Charles Revson, his two brothers, and Charles Lachman formed Revlon in 1932 as a nail polish manufacturer. Before the Revlon venture, Charles Lachman was connected by marriage to a company that manufactured nail enamel. Charles Revson had worked for two years selling nail polish produced by another company called Elka. Elka's nail polish was unusual for its time. Competing products typically were made with dyes; they were transparent and limited to three shades of red. The Elka product was opaque. Revson believed such a product in a wide range of shades could capture the market. When Elka management dismissed his ideas, Revson left and founded Revlon. Sales growth was spectacular—from $4,000 in 1932 to $606 million in 1974, Revson's last year in charge.

In 1940, Revlon added lipstick to its product line in an advertising campaign called "Matching Lips and Finger Tips." It featured Revlon's first full-color, two-page ads. During the 1940s, Revlon's marketing continued to tie cosmetic color to fashion. Each spring and fall, it announced new colors, and Revson gave each of them attractive and evocative names. For example, the 1945 color was "Fatal Apple." "Plumb Beautiful" was the shade of 1949. "Where's The Fire" was the key shade and theme for 1950. "Fire and Ice," which appeared in 1952, was Revson's biggest promotional success. Each of these annual promotional events were supported with every form of media available at the time. Revlon was one of the first of the modern cosmetics companies to sponsor its own television shows ("The $64,000 Question") and to develop its own celebrity spokesperson (the Revlon girls of the 1950s were as famous as the Rockettes).

THE PRODUCT MUST DELIVER

The primary benefits sought in a nail polish brand are:

- Offers a variety of colors.
- Provides a glossy shine.
- Doesn't "chip."
- Dries quickly.

Each of these represents the high road for potential brand positionings.

POSITIONING EXAMPLES

- Revlon's 1985 and 1995 launches of new improved products with longer lasting nail enamel formulations was built on an important secondary benefit ("not chipping"). Nevertheless, both new improved launches were successful enough to allow Revlon to retain its fifty-year leadership of the nail enamel segment (twenty-five share of market).[7]
- Chesebrough-Ponds' 1985 launch of the Aziza Nail Polish Pen is an example of a strong concept coupled (unfortunately) with a weak product. "The Pen" was the ultimate in simplicity— "paint your fingers with the same ease as coloring in a picture." There was only one problem—the product didn't work (it clogged after one use and dried up). Because the concept was terrific, "The Pen" had great trial, but no repeat business—a lesson for every marketer.

THE LIPSTICK MARKET

The lipstick market accounted for approximately $1.3 billion in 1995 and was the fastest growing segment in cosmetics during the period 1993–1995.[8] This lipstick boom was fueled by the innovation of "long-wearing" formulas developed by Revlon in 1994 and driven by significant marketing support.

THE PRODUCT MUST DELIVER

Lipstick is a color-driven business. And so, having a wide variety of colors to choose from is the price of entry. Additionally, a lipstick now must have the additional characteristics of long wearing ("not having to reapply lipstick throughout the day") as well as moisturizing properties (protecting lips from chapping or drying).

POSITIONING EXAMPLES

- Revlon's ColorStay introduction in 1994 solved the most important problem of lipstick users—how to make lipstick last longer ("women *hate* reapplying lipstick throughout the day"). Revlon's share increased from twenty-seven to thirty-five in one year after this introduction.[9]
- L'Oreal's 1995 Color Endure Lipstick also had a long-lasting benefit, as well as a purportedly better moisturizing formula. By combining long lasting with a formulation that combats dryness, L'Oreal delivered a big consumer benefit—it married two price of entry benefits together.
- Coty's 1995 launch of Hold It was built on lessons learned from skin care marketing. Hold It is a product that is applied before a woman puts on her lipstick. Offering the benefit of better adhesion, this introduction was interesting because it built on a woman's propensity to use a "regimen" of products. This transference of technology (from skin care to cosmetics)

Marketing Cosmetics **99**

can be an important means for successfully marketing beauty care products.

All of these innovations were done within the context of the category's basic mass price points, and so, they reinforced the value-added nature of these products. Neither Revlon nor L'Oreal raised their price points when they brought out their new improved formulations.

FACIAL MAKEUP

The overwhelming desire of Boomers (particularly the Mature Stylists) to retard the aging process has been the driving force in facial makeup throughout the 1990s.

THE PRODUCT MUST DELIVER

Facial makeup must contain some anti-aging ingredient as well as provide a natural skin tone base that has the ability to conceal facial imperfections.

POSITIONING EXAMPLES

- Revlon's 1994 launch of Age Defying Makeup revolutionized the category. Suddenly, anti-aging properties became price of entry requirements. Revlon's sales increased nearly thirty percent the first year after this introduction.[10] Revlon's strategy keyed not only on the demographics of the Boomers, but was clearly targeted to those Boomers who classified themselves as Mature Stylists. The advertising campaign, "Defy Your Age," featuring actress Melanie Griffith, conveyed this message with quiet yet defiant class.
- Cover Girl, the category leader with a thirty share of market (which has been maintained throughout the 1990s), also has consistently innovated.[11] Its 1995 launch of Balanced

Complexion Liquid Makeup was nearly as revolutionary as Revlon's Age Defying Makeup. Balanced Complexion Liquid Makeup was the first major facial cosmetic product specifically geared to consumers who have partly oily and partly dry skin (termed combination skin in the cosmetic business). This new technology, which delivered moisturizing benefits to dry areas while controlling shine in oily ones, created a new price of entry benefit—improving combination skin.

- Maybelline's positioning of its 1995 launch of Revitalizing Makeup is nearly identical to Revlon's. The primary difference is the target group. Maybelline's message is skewed significantly younger than Revlon's (Maybelline = Xers, Revlon = Boomers). Maybelline has further refined Xers by appealing to those that classify themselves as Impressionists. This dedication to "market fragmentation" (see Chapter 3) is largely responsible for Maybelline's long-term success.

EYE MAKEUP

Eye makeup must fill one of three uses:

- **Anti-aging.** Most importantly, eye makeup must cover up one of the first signs of aging—"crows feet" (the slight wrinkles around the eyes).
- **Matches consumer's eye color.** The consumer desires to match the color of her eyes with eye makeup to enhance her beauty. The goal is to make the eyes literally "the window of the soul." The eyes become the focal point of the consumer's being (a la Elizabeth Taylor).
- **Matches consumer's wardrobe.** A wide variety of colors enable the consumer to match eye makeup to the color of the clothes she is wearing.

A Case Study

MAYBELLINE

Maybelline has been the undisputed leader in the eye makeup category since 1915. The brief recap below of Maybelline's beginnings and continuing emphasis on innovation are lessons that every marketer should learn. This synopsis was taken from Bud Brewster's "50 Years of Cosmetic Color" (an article written in December 1995 for Cosmetics and Toiletries).

- T.L. Williams, the founder of Maybelline (which was named after his sister Mabel), believed in the power of advertising and promotion.[12] Maybelline was the first cosmetic advertiser on radio and television.[13] In the 1940s, actresses Hedy Lamar and Joan Crawford promoted the product; in the 1980s, it was TV's Wonder Woman, Linda Carter; and in the 1990s, it's model Christy Turlington.[14]

- Maybelline has invested in research and development to maintain its dominance in eye makeup. Maybelline was one of the first cosmetic companies to implement hypoallergenic testing; it also was among the first to add sunscreen protection. Additionally, Maybelline was the first to claim contact lens compatibility for all its mascaras.[15]

- Maybelline's 1995 launch of Lash by Lash Mascara demonstrates the marketer's continued commitment to innovation through real product improvements. Although the benefit of Lash by Lash is based on a secondary benefit ("no clumping"), it's still using high technology to solidify its overall leadership position in eye makeup.

POSITIONING EXAMPLE

- L'Oreal's 1995 launch of Voluminous Waterproof Mascara technologically takes on Maybelline's Lash By Lash. Voluminous Waterproof uses a co-polymer complex originally

COSMETIC SEGMENT SUMMARY: KEY BENEFITS AND DRIVERS

	LIPSTICK	NAIL ENAMEL	EYE MAKEUP	FACIAL MAKEUP
Primary Drivers (Price of Entry Elements)	Available in wide variety of colors	Comes in wide variety of colors	Covers "crow's feet"	Available in wide variety of colors
	Moisturizes lips	Provides high shine	Matches natural color of eyes	Retards aging process (look younger)
	Lasts through the day		Matches color of clothes	Offers formulations for different skin types
			Matches color of skin tones	Conceals facial imperfections
Secondary Drivers (Absence of Negatives)	Colors evenly	Dries quickly	Hypoallergenic	Prevents shine
	Goes on smoothly	Doesn't chip	Doesn't clump	Lasts all day
	Offers sun protection		Lasts through the day	Hypoallergenic

developed for hairspray and transfers that technology to eye makeup.[16] Although "waterproof" is only a secondary benefit (like "no clumping"), it's high on the consumer's list of important eye makeup features. Also the transference of technology (from hair care to cosmetics) makes a more easily understood story for the consumer.

Chapter 7

MARKETING SKIN CARE

MARKET DYNAMICS

IN 1995, THE OVERALL SKIN CARE MARKET topped $4.4 billion.[17] This represents nearly a thirty percent growth rate over the previous five years.[18] It is estimated that, by the end of this century, the skin care market will be $5.3 billion. The primary segments that constitute the skin care market are hand and body lotions, facial treatments (moisturizers and cleansers), sun care, and bath and liquid cleansing products.

The manufacturers that dominate skin care are the heavy duty hitters of packaged goods: L'Oreal, Unilever, Procter & Gamble, Shering-Plough, S.C. Johnson, Warner Lambert, Bristol Myers, Estee Lauder, and Revlon. These companies have considerable resources and invest in research and development, advertising, and operations.

1995 SKIN CARE SEGMENT IMPORTANCE

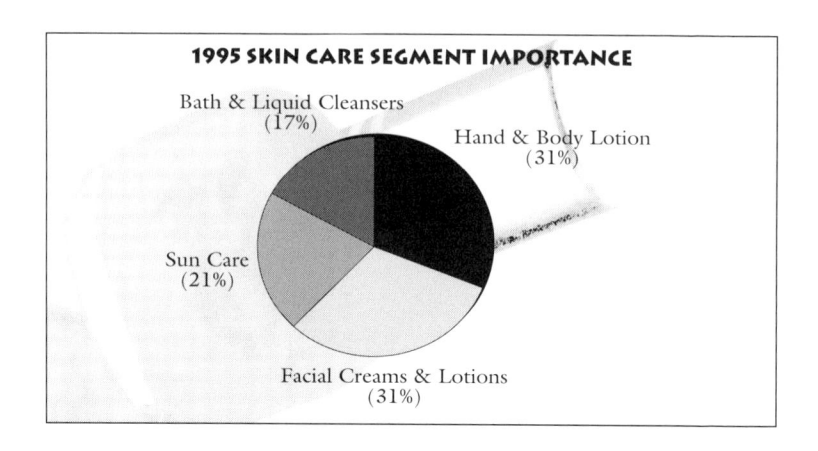

- Bath & Liquid Cleansers (17%)
- Hand & Body Lotion (31%)
- Sun Care (21%)
- Facial Creams & Lotions (31%)

HAND AND BODY LOTIONS

At $1.4 billion, the hand and body lotion market is one of the largest segments in personal care ($780 million in the food/drug/mass classes of trade; $580 million in the prestige/direct marketing classes of trade).[19] Seventy percent of adult women use a hand and body lotion daily.[20] Such high usage is driven by the real and perceived belief that they have dry skin (more than eighty-five percent of adult women believe that they have dry skin; more than a third believe that they have rough or chapped skin).[21]

Body lotions have one of the fastest consumption rates of any personal care products (repurchase takes place between six and eight weeks). Consumers use up body lotions so quickly because they are applied extensively over the body: arms, legs, elbows, knees, feet, heels, face, neck, breasts, and stomach. This category will continue to get attention from marketers because of its extensive and frequent use after many mundane tasks (after showering, washing dishes, and doing house chores and before going out and going to bed).

POSITIONING EXAMPLES

Unilever's Vaseline Intensive Care Lotion has been the number one brand in food, drug, and mass merchandisers since its introduction in 1971. This twenty-five year dominance of the category is a function of the brand consistently being dedicated to its therapeutic positioning which promises both "healing and moisturizing" benefits (the two primary price of entry benefits sought after in a hand and body lotion).

- The positioning of Vaseline Intensive Care Lotion is supported with a continued commitment to improving the basic product proposition. At least once every three years a "new improved" formulation is brought forward. In addition, Unilever also is committed to "new news" by way of different line extensions (Sensitive Skin, Extra Strength, etc.). The brand is then consistently supported with a media program averaging between $8 million–$12 million. This represents about a six to eight percent advertising to sales ratio each and every year.

A Case Study

P&G WONDRA HAND LOTION

Companies that have attempted to develop new hand and body lotions based on secondary positionings ("not being greasy" for example) have not been successful. The most dramatic failure was Procter & Gamble's Wondra in the late 1970s. Although Wondra's demise occurred twenty years ago, the lessons for marketers are as salient today as they were then.

- Procter & Gamble targeted the hand and body lotion market for nearly a decade prior to the introduction of Wondra. It was the only major category in personal care or beauty care that was not represented by a dominant Procter & Gamble brand. Procter & Gamble (as it has done throughout its corporate life) went to school on the lotion category. It knew that an efficacious formulation with great moisturizing properties was critical for success. After completing extensive product testing, Procter & Gamble introduced a very thick moisturizing formula. In fact, it was so thick that it required a revolutionary dispenser—the upside down bottle (otherwise the lotion would settle at the bottom and clog a traditional "right-side" up container). Procter & Gamble viewed the dispenser as a means for creating interest and a "point of difference" (someone should have warned them about being careful what you wish for).

- Consumers found the dispenser to be such a departure from the norm, that they would forget that the spout side had to be put face down after use. Thus, the consumer had a tendency to put it "face-up" (like every other product in beauty care). When this occurred, the bottle would tip over causing a "domino effect" in their medicine cabinet, closet, night stand, or drawer.
- The trade also had trouble with the container. Procter & Gamble had demanded end aisle displays for Wondra during its roll-out period. Store personnel constantly were standing the bottle the wrong way creating havoc at the store level. The displays kept falling (they looked like bowling pins in a bowling alley). Further, consumers who picked up a bottle in the store and then placed it back on the shelf also created a problem for in-store personnel—the shelves of hand lotions required constant maintenance. **Lesson: The most difficult element to change is buyer behavior. The "upside down" bottle required a change in behavior from consumers. The change was not forthcoming, and the product failed.**
- Beyond the dispenser, Procter & Gamble chose to make the "non-greasy" aspect of Wondra's formulation its primary positioning element. "Non-greasy" is a secondary benefit (an absence of a negative) rather than a primary benefit. It was

not nearly as persuasive as a moisturizing/healing platform (as in the case of Vaseline Intensive Care Lotion). Within a few short years, Procter & Gamble withdrew Wondra from the shelves. It was one of the few failures in Procter & Gamble's history.

On the class side of the business, Estee Lauder's 1996 introduction of "Thigh Zone Body Streamlining Complex" is an excellent example of introducing a successful body lotion. Estee Lauder's positioning was based on a proven marketing technique—the problem/solution approach.

- "Thigh Zone" played to a problem which already had acquired significant notoriety—cellulite. The advertising headlines focused on "scientific news": "New knowledge uncovers the real causes of cellulite. And a real answer."
- Estee Lauder's advertising set up the skin care product manufacturer as an authority in the field. "Now there's new technology from Estee Lauder Research to deal with the problem. Thigh Zone."
- Perhaps the most important element of the Estee Lauder product was the fact that Thigh Zone was used in the same way consumers used body lotions (pouring from a bottle onto the hands and then spreading on the skin area). Thus, although purporting to be a new product, it did not ask the consumer to change her behavior. Estee Lauder recognized that changing consumer behavior was a long, drawn-out process—and a costly one.
- Further, by playing to "thighs," Estee Lauder was the beneficiary of large advertising campaigns directed at this body area by hosiery manufacturers. Whether it was Sara Lee's spokespersons Fran Dressler, Jamie Lee Curtis, or Tina Turner "selling" the benefits of "Smooth Silhouettes" or No nonsense's Sela Ward extolling "Great Shapes," there was no doubt that Estee Lauder

benefited from the added emphasis that both of these manufacturers placed against "thigh control." **Lesson: Look to the categories where a similar problem/solution approach is being discussed and determine if there is an opportunity to "tag along."**

FACIAL MOISTURIZERS

The facial moisturizer segment accounts for nearly $900 million.[22] More than seventy percent of women use a facial moisturizer at least a couple of times a week, and fifty percent use a facial moisturizer at least once a day.[23]

Anti-wrinkling and anti-aging claims dominate most marketers' efforts. This is a category that requires patience on the part of manufacturers, if they are to be successful, because the facial moisturizer segment generally has long purchase cycles and, therefore, is a slow build in the marketplace. The marketing investment is considerable; it requires consistent advertising support and trial generating vehicles, which are always expensive.

It is for this reason that the payoff for this category generally is long term (at least three to four years). **The good news is, once you've developed a user base, they tend to remain loyal. Remember, few categories are as emotionally charged as face care; the face is the first battleground where women wage war against the aging process. Thus, consumers are cautious about changing products and/or trying new ones.** The "risk" is enormous both from an emotional standpoint as well as an economic one; most facial moisturizing products are fairly expensive—even those purchased in the mass market channels.

The primary ingredient for the 1990s has been the proliferation of Alpha Hydroxy Acid products (AHAs). AHAs are the "hope in a bottle" for the '90s, and their popularity will continue to grow as long as tests purport that these exfoliants work in minimizing the signs of aging.[24] Further, they also offer the ecological elements consumers want, since they are derived from fruits and other natural substances.[25]

POSITIONING EXAMPLES

Success in facial moisturizers is virtually contingent on providing anti-wrinkling or anti-aging claims. L'Oreal's Plenitude in 1988 made anti-aging the price of entry in the category. It proved that a unique ingredient "liposomes" served up with "scientific proof" is an excellent formula for success ("liposomes" has since become a common word in beauty care ingredient formulations).

- In launching Plenitude, L'Oreal also wrote the book on what is required from an advertising and promotion standpoint to successfully market a facial moisturizer. The key to Plenitude's success was product sampling. **Lesson: In the case of a new product category segment, advertising alone will not successfully convert enough triers without an additional (and extensive) in-home sampling effort.**

Plenitude's most important contribution was that it made other marketers such as Procter & Gamble, Colgate, and Unilever realize that U.S. consumers were ready for more sophisticated skin care products.

- Nivea's 1995 introduction of Visage Optimale Cumulative Care Creme scored effectively with the consumer. It combines the number one price of entry benefit (the promise of "looking younger") with the ultimate payoff—"instantly improved results." The concept was then further enhanced with an additional "guarantee" that "results will get better the longer you use the product."
- L'Oreal's Revitalift Firming Creme targets its message to older Boomers. It's squarely positioned to Mature Stylists within the Boomer generation. The ability of L'Oreal to effectively

segment its consumer base between Older Boomers (Revitalizing Firming Creme) and Younger Boomers (Plenitude) is a critical reason why L'Oreal has retained its number one ranking in beauty care worldwide dollar sales.[26]

- Unilever's Pond's brand has been able to turn its business around through the magic ingredient of the '90s—Alpha Hydroxy Acid (AHA). Coupling this anti-aging ingredient with a strong marketing program has spelled success for Pond's. A critical part of this "make-over" for Pond's was the selection of a name. **Pond's Age Defying Moisturizer is an excellent example of how a name can be synonymous with a call to action. Can there be a more action oriented word than "defy"?**

- Another way to gain a stronghold in the facial moisturizer category is to expand body usage. Mary Kay's Skin Revival System was positioned for face and throat. As the population ages, the throat will get more attention.

- **"Ease of use" has always been a route to success.** Maybelline's Alpha Hydroxy Intensive Night Creme is a good example of how this works for a beauty care product. The promise of "waking up to better results" is a powerful aphrodisiac, particularly for Mature Stylists.

FACIAL CLEANSERS

The facial cleanser market is nearly $600 million due to thirty-nine percent of households using a facial cleanser daily.[27] It also is a proliferated category: In 1994, more than 150 new facial cleansing products were introduced (this includes, new products, line extensions, new sizes, etc.).

The facial cleanser segment tends to be driven more by product performance than by emotional claims. Facial cleansers have a bimodal skew: Both younger and older women use these products; yet they are looking for different types of "clean."

- Younger women want rinseable lotions that deep clean the pores.
- Older women are more apt to use a cleanser with a cream that removes makeup and/or is a non-drying alternative to soap.

POSITIONING EXAMPLES

- Noxema, a brand leader for two decades, still does a great job of contemporizing its product, while providing the necessary claims and reassurances that make it nearly a "timeless" item. Its overall headline "Great Face" is the end goal for all cleanser and cosmetic and skin care users. Noxema's dual promise to "deep clean" coupled with "conditions too" supports the payoff of "leaves your face looking and feeling healthy."
- St. Ives' 1995 Vanilla and Honey Facial Wash introduction helped pioneer a relatively new price of entry benefit in facial cleansers—nourishment and cleaning. The concept of "dual benefits" is certainly common enough in beauty care products, but relatively new in facial cleansers. St. Ives took a page from hair care (where vanilla as well as other natural ingredients are purported to provide nourishment to the hair roots) and brought it to skin care. Over and over again, we see that **the ability to transfer technology from one beauty care category to another can be a tremendous avenue for growth.**
- Procter & Gamble's Oil of Olay 1995 introduction of "Facial Wash" extends Olay's moisturizing expertise into the cleansing arena. This product's promise to "retard cellular aging" as well as cleanse continues to be a potent means for positioning facial cleansers. Again, the bundling of dual benefits and the transference of technology has proven to be a success.

SUN CARE

The sun care market was more than $500 million in 1995.[28] This represents more than a thirty-five percent increase since 1991. Market growth has been driven by the growing awareness and acceptance of the dangers of the sun. This has led to an ever-increasing level of SPF (Sun Protection Factors) products in the marketplace. In 1986, sun care products with SPF levels of over 15 accounted for only ten percent of sun protection sales. Today more than sixty percent of sun care products have SPF levels over 15.[29]

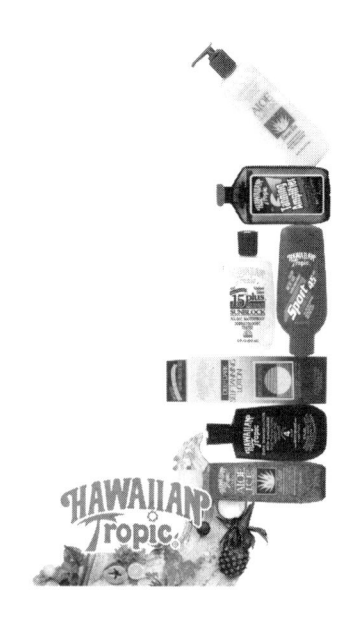

POSITIONING EXAMPLE

- Hawaiian Tropics has done a good job of capturing the primary characteristics desired in a sun care product—protection and rejuvenation. It offers "gentle formulas that have less chemicals

SKIN CARE SEGMENT SUMMARY: KEY BENEFITS AND DRIVERS

	HAND & BODY LOTIONS	FACIAL MOISTURIZERS	FACIAL CLEANSERS	SUN CARE	BATH & LIQUID CLEANSERS
Primary Drivers (Price of Entry Elements)	Makes skin soft & smooth	Makes facial skin soft & smooth	Cleans skin	Protects against sunburn, wrinkling, cancer	Cleanses
	Heals dry/chapped skin	Prevents wrinkling	Removes makeup		Relaxes
	Prevents dry skin	Makes user look younger	Reduces moisture loss	Allows sunless tanning	Moisturizes & cleanses
Secondary Drivers (Absence of Negatives)	Isn't greasy	Contains natural ingredients	Offers non-drying formulation	Hypoallergenic	Offers non-drying formulation
	Absorbs	Hypoallergenic		Long lasting	
		Absorbs quickly		Water-proof	
		Be non-greasy		Be non-greasy	
				All family usage	

Marketing Skin Care

than before—yet offer better protection," as well as "time-released Vitamins A, C, and E to fight signs of photo-aging." The use of time-released ingredients infers "scientific proof" for why the product works. The fact that Hawaiian Tropics has different formulations for children and adults is further support for the trade to provide the brand with additional shelf space. This is "strong marketing" that gives Hawaiian Tropics a real point of difference in the marketplace.

BATH AND LIQUID BODY CLEANSERS

In 1995, the total bath and liquid body cleanser category totaled $750 million (with approximately sixty percent of the dollars being generated by products sold in food, drug, and discount stores).[30] The liquid body cleanser segment accounts for nearly three-quarters of the retail sales in the "mass" class of trade.[31] It is one of the fastest growing categories in all of beauty care. This category has nearly doubled in size in less than three years.[32]

A Case Study
JERGENS SHOWER-ACTIVE
KAO's Jergens was the innovative market leader in the liquid body cleanser segment. In 1994, Jergens launched its successful Jergens Body Shampoo and, in late fall 1995, introduced Shower Active. In both cases, Jergens targeted not the seventeen percent of households that used bath products, but rather the seventy-five percent of women who claim to have "dry skin."[33]

Shower Active is almost the prototypical type of product that will be needed in skin care in the future. In creating this product, Jergens used new technology in an effort to protect and treat extremely dry skin. Jergens came up with a clear (to give the consumer a sense of purity), water-activated polymer/gel formula that worked on wet skin, when skin is at its moisturizing peak.[34] From a marketing vantage point, Jergens went to school on the consumer.

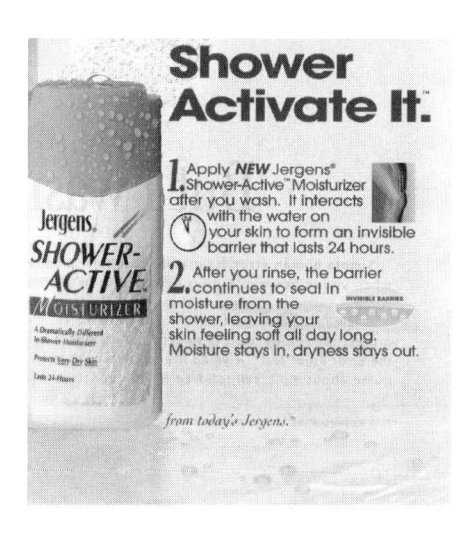

Shower Activate It.

1. Apply *NEW* Jergens® Shower-Active™ Moisturizer after you wash. It interacts with the water on your skin to form an invisible barrier that lasts 24 hours.

2. After you rinse, the barrier continues to seal in moisture from the shower, leaving your skin feeling soft all day long. Moisture stays in, dryness stays out.

from today's Jergens.

Jergens' research showed that the usual method of applying lotion after a shower or bath was considered too time consuming by the majority of its test respondents. Shower Active addressed this need by allowing the consumer to quickly and easily treat dry skin by applying a moisturizer in the shower. This built on the behavior already exhibited by women: Virtually all women regularly shave their legs in the shower and then moisturize them. In extensive product testing the consumer's voice said it all: "This product made my skin silky after just one use. I like the easy way you can use it, the fragrance was good, and it made my skin smooth and moisturized."[35]

Chapter 8

MARKETING HAIR CARE PRODUCTS

MARKET DYNAMICS: CATEGORY SIZE AND SEGMENT IMPORTANCE

IF WE START WITH THE PREMISE that "no matter what, a woman wants her hair to look good,"[36] then it is not surprising to note that the hair care market had a retail dollar volume level of nearly $6 billion in 1995 making it by far the largest beauty care segment in the mass market.[37] Although shampoos and conditioners account for the largest share of the dollars, sizable businesses are noted for hairspray, hair coloring, styling aids (mousses, gels, spritzes), home permanents, and ethnic hair care products.

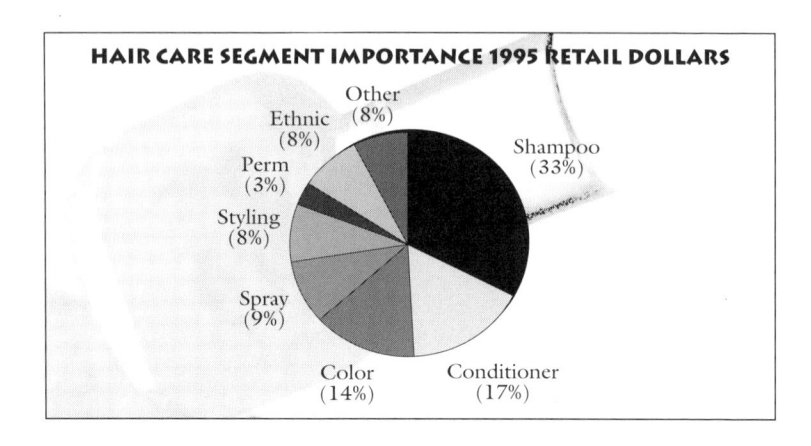

HAIR CARE SEGMENT IMPORTANCE 1995 RETAIL DOLLARS

- Shampoo (33%)
- Conditioner (17%)
- Color (14%)
- Spray (9%)
- Styling (8%)
- Perm (3%)
- Ethnic (8%)
- Other (8%)

No other beauty care category embodies the amount of "fragmentation" as the hair care category. Further, it is the only beauty care segment that does nearly eighty percent of its dollar volume in the food, drug, or mass merchandiser trade channels; it is estimated that less than two percent of all the dollars are contributed by the traditional prestige sector (the department store trade class).[38] In the case of hair care, the outlet for "prestige" products is the salon channel. This outlet for hair care includes both beauty salons as well as professional beauty care product shops selling only professional products.

MARKET DYNAMICS: CATEGORY USAGE AND PRODUCT SEGMENTATION

Usage is high across all segments. Ninety percent of households use a shampoo regularly (once a week or more often), eighty percent used a conditioner in the past month (includes combination products), fifty percent regularly use hairspray, forty-five percent use some type of styling aid, and fifty-two percent use some form of a hair coloring agent (includes multipurpose products such as shampoos containing a color enhancer).[39]

From both a consumer segmentation and product point of view, this is a category built on the premise that "more is better than less." Therefore, within each of the primary segments, there are a myriad of subsegments and specialty products:

- **Products for specific hair types:** normal, dry, oily, and combination hair.
- **Products for processed hair:** permed or color-treated.
- **Products for particular conditions:** dry scalp and dandruff, hair strengtheners, body builders, and detanglers.
- **Products to stimulate different consumer sensory preferences:** variations in strength or type of fragrances (in order to connote different feelings); all natural products (shampoos and conditioners primarily); form variations (liquids, gels, or concentrates; sprays or spritzes; pumps or aerosols; tubes, jars, or bottles); and color preferences (light to dark, blondes to brunettes).

MARKET DYNAMICS: KEY PLAYERS AND STRATEGIES

In assessing the key manufacturers in hair care, it is a formidable list: **Procter & Gamble** (Pert, Head and Shoulders, Pantene, Vidal Sassoon, Prell, and Ivory); **Unilever** (Rave hair care products, Aqua Net, Faberge Organics, and the Helene Curtis products: Suave, Finesse, Salon Selectives); **Bristol Myers' Clairol Division** (Herbal Essence, Nice 'N Easy, Loving Care, Condition); **L'Oreal** (Preference, Studio Line, Castings, Accenting); **Gillette** (White Rain hair care products and Silkience hair care lines); **Johnson and Johnson** (Neutrogena and J&J Baby Shampoo); and **Revlon** (Flex and Realistic ethnic hair products).

One axiom dominates each of these successful companies—they are committed to hair care. To truly understand this commitment, you must understand the two common characteristics that each of these companies possesses:

- **Each company has a multitude of brand names and extends these brand names into several different hair care categories.** The net result is that each brand has a distinctly carved out image that stands separately from the parent company (for example, Vidal Sassoon from Procter & Gamble). Thus, the overall brand trademark (Vidal Sassoon) acts as a source of authority as well as a "guarantee" of product performance.
- **The companies further differentiate each of their brands through price/benefit oriented positioning platforms and link each brand to different consumer segments.** The blending of price/benefit and consumer orientation is fused together through a balance of functional performance characteristics as well as emotional cues (see the examples that follow for shampoos and conditioners).

The following charts recap the primary hair care companies, their brands, principal positioning characteristics, and key segments that they are targeted against.

In addition to having a multitude of brands in their stables (each with a different positioning), these manufacturers are aggressive in their marketing efforts. These efforts encompass:

- Periodic commitments to restagings via new improved formulations and updated packaging and graphics.
- Continued introductions of line extensions (at least once every twelve to eighteen months).
- Ongoing media support (advertising-to-sales ratios tend to run at the ten percent level for brand segment leaders).

EXAMPLES OF COMPANIES WITH A MULTI-SEGMENT AND MULTI-BENEFIT APPROACH TO HAIR CARE

COMPANY	BRAND	SEGMENT	POSITIONING	SEGMENT ORIENTATION
Procter & Gamble	Ivory	Price/Value	"Pure Clean"	Fundamentalists
	Prell	Price/Value	"Convenience"	Traditionalists
	Head & Shoulders	Premium-Specialty	Multifunctional: cleanses & removes dandruff	Broad-based appeal; however, skewed to Fundamentalists & Traditionalists
	Pert Plus	Premium-Specialty	Cleans & conditions	Broad-based appeal: however, skewed to Fundamentalists & Traditionalists
	Pantene Pro V	Prestige	Ultra-mild product: Complete opposite of multifunctional products; geared to fully cleanse hair of other agents	Mature Stylists & Impressionists
	Vidal Sassoon	Prestige	Salon Heritage	Appeals to both Mature Stylists & Impressionists

Marketing Hair Care Products

EXAMPLES OF COMPANIES WITH A MULTI-SEGMENT AND MULTI-BENEFIT APPROACH TO HAIR CARE

COMPANY	BRANDS	SEGMENT	POSITIONING	SEGMENT ORIENTATION
Helene Curtis (Unilever)	Suave	Price/Value	"Smart Shopper"	Appeals almost equally to Fundamentalists & Traditionalists
	Finesse	Premium	"Product Is Hero": technological orientation (self-adjusting)	Aimed at both Traditionalists & Mature Stylists
	Salon Selectives	Premium	"Have It Your Way": purchaser in control (consumer has choice of four conditioning levels)	Appeal aimed at youthful end of Impressionists & Mature Stylists segments
L'Oreal	Colorvive	Premium-Specialty/Protection	Technological orientation; ultraviolet filter to protect color-treated hair	Mature Stylist
	Preference	Premium	"I'm Worth It": inner-directed; permanent hair coloring	Appeals to both Mature Stylists & Impressionists
	Castings	Moderate Price Point	Technological orientation; safety; temporary hair coloring—easy entry point	Broad-based appeal: Traditionalists, Mature Stylists & Impressionists
	Accenting	Premium	Technological orientation; safety; highlights hair (vs. colors hair)	Broad-based appeal to consumers interested in accenting current hair color; further segmented by the fact that it is made primarily for women with dark hair
	Studio Line	Moderate Price Point	Encourages style creativity; youthful orientation	Appeals primarily to youthful end of Impressionist segment

EXAMPLES OF COMPANIES WITH A MULTI-SEGMENT AND MULTI-BENEFIT APPROACH TO HAIR CARE

COMPANY	BRAND	SEGMENT	POSITIONING	SEGMENT ORIENTATION
Clairol (Bristol Myers)	Herbal Essence	Moderate Price Point	Natural orientation: "environmentally safe"	Broad-based appeal across segments: aimed at consumers interested in natural products
	Glints	Moderate Price Point	Multipurpose semi-permanent hair color; conditions and colors; emotional safety—easy entry point for consumers interested in hair coloring but afraid of either damaging hair or long-term effects if they don't like the results	Broad-based appeal: Traditionalists, Mature Stylists & Impressionists
	Nice 'N Easy	Moderate Price Point	Permanent hair color	Mature Stylists & Traditionalists

THE FUTURE OF HAIR CARE

Hair care products (particularly shampoos and conditioners) will continue to keep coming out, but few will achieve lasting success. (Pert 2-1 is the only hair care product introduced since 1980 to ever achieve and maintain a double digit unit and dollar share of market.) The reason is simple—the promise of a new shampoo or conditioner that purports new or better benefits presents a great temptation for the consumer because the risk of failure is relatively small (unlike using a face care or cosmetics product). **Marketers may successfully maintain brand franchises by transferring skin care and cosmetic technologies into proprietary hair care products.**

POSITIONING EXAMPLES: SHAMPOOS AND CONDITIONERS

L'Oreal's 1995 introduction of performance shampoos is an excellent example of the trend of taking advantage of breakthroughs in technology, particularly skin care.[40] Savvy L'Oreal gained additional shelf space by positioning each variant against a different "scientific" dimension. From a retailer's perspective, L'Oreal offered the consumer non-duplicative alternatives that merited more incremental shelf space.

- Fortavive Performance Shampoo was designed to replace the ceramide naturally found in the hair, but lost every day. Ceramides are the complex lipids found between the layers of the hair's cuticle scales that protect the inner structure of the hair.
- Colorvive Shampoo incorporates a patented ultraviolet filter to protect color-treated hair.
- Hydravive Shampoo restores moisture to dry hair due to a protein complex consisting of a hygroscopic ingredient derived from natural wheat.

"Natural" shampoos and conditioners made a strong comeback in the '90s. However, the consumer of the '90s has a "strong taste for sorting out what works and what doesn't, compared to the consumer who bought shampoos containing everything from blueberries to eggs in the early '70s."[41] **The primary reason that naturals, particularly botanical additives, are becoming increasingly popular with manufacturers and retailers is that the more exotic the botanical ingredient the more expensive it becomes; this adds "significantly to the sticker price" thereby fattening the margins.**[42] The key with all of the exotic ingredients is that they have to work.

- Matrix Essentials (one of the leading salon brands) uses *chitosan*, a "renewal resource" from the African rain forest. It is purported to protect the hair and help it hold a set or a straightened style.[43]

POSITIONING EXAMPLES: HAIR COLORING PRODUCTS

The '90s saw an explosion in the women's hair coloring market; it was the only hair care sector to record double digit growth levels from 1993–1995. "Over half of all women are coloring their hair. This is particularly true among baby boomers. Research shows that baby boomers tend to see themselves as youthful and never growing old. Baby boomers are the most receptive to anti-aging strategies and are the most frequent users of hair coloring to hide gray."[45]

Beyond the Boomers, younger women (the Generation X crowd) also turned towards hair coloring products in the late '90s. "Hair has become an important fashion accessory for the younger woman who wants to enhance, brighten, or add drama to her natural pigmented hair."[46]

HAIR CARE SUMMARY: KEY BENEFITS AND DRIVERS

	SHAMPOO	CONDITIONERS	HAIR COLORING	STYLING AIDS (HAIRSPRAYS/MOUSSES/GELS)
Primary Drivers (Price of Entry elements)	Cleans hair	Makes hair healthy	Provides long lasting hair color	Holds a style
	Leaves hair looking healthy	Makes hair manageable	Provides temporary hair coloring	Provides a soft hold
	Gives hair body	Gives hair shine	Adds hair highlights	Makes hair easy to style
	Contains a dandruff additive	Makes hair stronger	Brightens natural hair color	Provides "wet look"
	Stops itching scalp	Makes hair easy to style		
	Gives hair shine	Self-adjusting conditioner		
	Restores hair moisture balance	Leave-in conditioner to produce soft hair		
	Protects color-treated hair			

128 *Beauty and the Beastly Market*

HAIR CARE SUMMARY: KEY BENEFITS AND DRIVERS

	SHAMPOO	CONDITIONERS	HAIR COLORING	STYLING AIDS (HAIRSPRAYS/MOUSSES/GELS)
	Won't leave hair feeling greasy	Won't leave hair feeling greasy	Conditions while coloring	Doesn't leave hair feeling stiff or sticky
	Available in a wide variety for different hair types	Available in a wide variety for different hair types	Won't damage hair	Won't harm hair
	Rinses out completely	Rinses out completely	Washes out after a few shampoos	Doesn't leave hair feeling greasy
	Made from natural products	Made from natural products	Won't burn scalp	Is easy to use
Secondary Drivers (Absence of Negatives)	Is part of a regimen system	Is part of a regimen system	Is quick & easy to use	

Marketing Hair Care Products

- Understanding that women were concerned about the lasting effects of permanent hair colorings, Clairol introduced Glints in early 1994. Glints was the first major semipermanent hair coloring product that had the benefits of accentuating a woman's natural hair color (adding subtle color tones, depth, and luster without substantially altering or damaging the natural hair).[47] Not only did Glints offer the "safety" of being semipermanent color (it washed out after six to eight shampooings), but it also only highlighted the hair's natural color. It also offered the reassurance of **no damage** because it contained no harsh chemicals (such as ammonia or peroxide). This secondary reassurance of "no damage" was an important element in Glints success.
- L'Oreal's Castings, introduced in late 1994, took Clairol's Glints one step further—it lasted up to six weeks (so it didn't have to be touched up as often). It too did not alter the natural pigment of the hair. Carol Hamilton, the executive vice president of L'Oreal for North America, summed up Castings in this manner: "Casting Tone-On-Tone Colorant is far and away the number one tone-on-tone in the marketplace. It is characterized as the most successful new hair color launch in a decade. It recognized a need women have for a gentler but longer-lasting hair color, particularly aging baby boomers."[48]
- Following the launch of Castings, Clairol introduced its own version of a longer-lasting, semipermanent color called Natural Instincts (in early 1995). It too was in tune with the times in that it was made with a combination of natural, botanical-based ingredients derived from pure sources.[49] "Natural Instincts is unique in its ability to deliver the conditioning benefits today's savvy consumers demand. Women today are most interested in enhancing their image rather than altering their image. In keeping with this trend, they are seeking products that allow them to complement their natural beauty while

expressing their individuality. Natural Instincts was specifically conceived to fulfill that aspiration."[50]

POSITIONING EXAMPLES: STYLING AIDS (HAIRSPRAYS/MOUSSES/GELS)

Gels, mousses, and hairsprays all have their "roots" squarely planted in the hairstyles of the day—they are fashion driven. The "hot" product of the day changes as the styles and fashions change. As is true with both fragrances and cosmetics, imagery as created by the written word can transform a "staid product into a younger product with a high style image."[51] The following are examples of this type of product dimensionalization:

PRODUCT REVITALIZATION THROUGH WORDS	
Old=Tired	New=Revitalized
"Hairspray"	Spritz"
"Setting Gel"	"Styling Gel"
"Body"	"Volume"
"Shine"	"Luster"

Many styling products have also come to be through "serendipity." They are important to review, because they represent how "savvy" marketers can transform what appear to be "roadblocks" into opportunities.

HAIRSPRAY

In late 1979, Chesebrough-Ponds introduced the first "soft" hairspray called Rave. At first glance this may sound like a contradiction in terms since the number one benefit desired in a hairspray is "long-lasting superhold." The marketing of Rave Hairspray was a direct lift from the textbook success of Rave Home Permanent, which was introduced the year before. The development of the Rave hair care line says a lot about the impact of serendipity as well as the astuteness of marketers to recognize potential opportunities from less than initial successful ventures.

A Case Study
RAVE HAIR CARE LINE

All through the mid-1970s, Chesebrough-Ponds (the maker of Vaseline, Vaseline Intensive Care Lotion, Ponds, and Cutex) had wanted to enter the hair care market. However, Chesebrough-Ponds also knew that to be successful in a potent competitive environment, it needed to have a technologically advanced product. Most of its efforts centered on the conditioner market (because consumers had a built-in perception that conditioners were "good for the hair"). And so, Chesebrough-Ponds concentrated on "deep conditioning."

The company developed a deep conditioner product, but it had two major problems: It took twenty minutes to work, and it did not wash "clean" out of the hair after one shampooing. The product, however, produced beautifully soft, manageable hair. After many meetings between marketing and R&D, it was determined that this formulation had potential in the home permanent market. Until then, there had not been a major introduction in the home permanent market in nearly two decades.

The technological advantage of Rave Home Permanent was that it did not contain any harsh chemical ingredients. It also had no odor because there was no ammonia used. This was a huge selling point. However, because it did not contain some of the harsher ingredients found in competitive products, it also could not produce extremely "tight" curls nor could it last as long as the leading home permanents—Toni and Lilt (which owned seventy-five percent of the market between them).

It was here that the marketing department of Chesebrough-Ponds took over from R&D. It made each of those negatives a selling point. In this regard, Rave was responsible for the revolution in "soft curls" and the "soft" hair positioning platform. It also provided the ultimate "guarantee"—**you now don't have to be afraid of damaging your hair or irritating your scalp.** Rave further provided an additional confidence dimension in that it was odor free. Hence, as Rave's advertising touted, the "neighborhood" doesn't have to endure the smell of your home permanent. The success of Rave Home Permanent was phenomenal—it became the number one home permanent in six short months.

The television commercial used to introduce Rave Home Permanent also was a breakthrough. It was the first commercial that used two "color" mediums—black and white and color. The commercial opened in black and white (indicating the past) and then segued into color (introducing the present and future). This commercial garnered enormous interest. Although Chesebrough-Ponds spent less than $4 million in the first year (a small sum even in those days to launch a new hair care product), it drove brand awareness to forty percent (an enormously high level given the dollars expended). By the end of the first year, Rave had captured the number one position in the home permanent market (thirty share), dislodging the two perennial giants—Procter & Gamble's Lilt and Gillette's Toni.

The packaging for Rave also was unusual. Prior to Rave's introduction, all major hair care products featured pictures of beautiful women on the cover of the box. After extensive market research testing, Chesebrough-Ponds discovered that women not only found it difficult to relate to those images, but were actually angry at the manufacturers ("I know I'm never going to look like that"). And so, Rave's package showed only an artist's rendering of beautiful hair which created a silhouette of a woman's face. Women responded enthusiastically: "I like envisioning myself on this package." **Lesson: Since packaging is the most important form of advertising (because it is what is seen** day in and day out on the shelf), all packaging should receive the kind of attention that Chesebrough-Ponds gave Rave.

Rave Hairspray also was positioned directly at the "soft" hair segment. After six months in the market, it had secured a five share of the then nearly $350 million hairspray market. It was the biggest success of any first year entry in this category.

It should also be noted that "serendipity" doesn't just happen; it must be discovered. Discovery requires a talented, intuitive, creative management. The original Rave team has since gone on to great success. Robert Phillips, the president then of Cheseborough-Ponds' Health and Beauty Aid Division, is now the CEO of Cheseborough-Ponds. Joseph Campinell, the director of new products for Chesebrough during Rave's launch, is now the vice president and general manager of L'Oreal North America; Jack Smith, the group product manager became the vice president of marketing for Readers Digest; and Carol Hamilton, the product manager on Rave, is now the executive vice president of marketing for L'Oreal North America.

MOUSSES

Recognizing environmental concerns, the United States in 1979 became the first country in the world to ban chlorofluorocarbons (CFCs) from consumer products. Suddenly, R&D and marketing folks alike were given the task of reinventing hairsprays. As a result of this government directive, the pump segment of the hairspray market increased. It also gave rise to new products with new marketing twists.

L'Oreal gave birth to the hair styling mousse in 1980.[52] By 1985, L'Oreal's Freehold Mousse controlled forty percent of a $150 million segment. Mousse is a foam product (it looks like a light shave cream) that is dispensed from an aerosol can. The product didn't contain harmful flurorocarbons, and it had little alcohol to dry the hair. The foam is rubbed into the hair and produces a "soft hold." Its primary benefit and major point of difference versus traditional hairsprays was that it didn't leave the brittle feel of hairsprays or the greasy look of gels.[53]

One of the key reasons for the success of mousse was that it combined two important consumer benefits desired in every beauty care product—convenience and ease of use. These are as relevant benefits for the year 2000 as they were in the preceding three decades. Alan Mottus, a well-known beauty consultant, summed it up: "We live in a push-button society and people want less mess and more convenience. Mousse has suddenly created an entirely new way of looking at packaging in the health and beauty aids business."

GELS

Hair gels are not a new phenomenon. Old time setting gels such as Dippity-Do have been redefined from "setting gels" to "styling gels." These products appeal squarely to young Generation X consumers who are predominately in the Impressionist segment.[54] Gels clearly demonstrate that a "tired" product (such as setting gels) can be reenergized by a repositioning that has its "roots" tied to a modern and relevant consumer target.

The growth of the gel market in the late 1980s and early 1990s was a direct outgrowth of the success of mousses. Mousses allowed consumers to understand that there can be different forms of styling products. Consumers grew accustomed to using mousses and were now looking for even more different types of products that would allow them to make their hair perform as they wanted. **This element of "control" has been a potent force permeating nearly every beauty care segment. It is the most important psychographic force in beauty care marketing to women.**

Chapter 9

MARKETING WOMEN'S FRAGRANCES

MARKET DYNAMICS: CATEGORY SIZE AND SEGMENT IMPORTANCE

THE WOMEN'S FRAGRANCE MARKET was $3.3 billion in 1995.[55] Although growth has been sluggish (approximately six percent per annum between 1992–1995), introductions continue to pervade the marketplace. In 1994, there were more than ninety new women's fragrances introduced into the United States.[56]

The reason for the large number of entries is due to the allure of hitting upon a winner. The average contribution margin for an established fragrance (defined as being in the market for three years or more) is said to be more than thirty percent.

Despite the opportunity for significant rewards, the financial risks in launching a fragrance are huge. Introducing a fragrance is one of the most expensive marketing investments in beauty care (Estee Lauder's Spellbound and Calvin Klein's Escape each cost

WOMEN'S FRAGRANCE SUMMARY: KEY BENEFITS AND DRIVERS

	TRADITIONAL FRAGRANCES	DESIGNER FRAGRANCES	UNISEX FRAGRANCES
Primary Drivers (Price of Entry characteristics)	Makes consumer feel feminine	Price validates who the consumer is	For people so secure they can share anything
	Is long lasting	Makes consumer feel feminine	Light/transparent scent
	Is a quality brand	Is long lasting	Clean/pure scent
	Promises happiness, freedom, & celebration in being a woman	Celebrates power, money, luxury, sex	
Secondary Drivers (Absence of Negatives)	Bottle must stand out	Exploit profitable synergy between fashion & perfume	Bottle must have utilitarian look
	Will make a suitable gift		Scent can't be overpowering
	Priced in $40-$50 range		

in the neighborhood of $25 million in advertising expenditures in the first year).[57] In the second year, advertising expenditures usually run about seventy-five percent of Year 1 levels, and in the third year, about fifty percent. A new fragrance brand doesn't begin to return its investment until its fourth year on the market (advertising then is only about thirty percent of the first year's advertising levels).

MARKET DYNAMICS: FRAGRANCE USAGE

Eighty-five percent of women use a perfume regularly; fifty percent put on a perfume or toilet water at least once a day.[58] **Women believe that "the perfume she wears says as much about how she sees herself and wants others to perceive her as her haircut or car."**[59] This is the reason so many women use fragrances.

In selecting a fragrance, there are a myriad of attitudes that come into play, but the most important is that "it makes a woman feel feminine." Beyond this one overriding characteristic, other selling points include the long-lasting nature of the scent, the brand name, the designer status, and whether it comes with a gift with purchase.

POSITIONING EXAMPLES

GIO

The 1993 Gio launch by L'Oreal confirms that even in a category as emotionally charged as fragrances, a classical approach to "the business of marketing" can pay off.

- L'Oreal's strategic objective for Gio was to develop a designer fragrance for the '90s—an era that was exemplified by classic and understated elegance (as opposed to the opulence of the

'80s). L'Oreal selected Armani because it believed "Georgio Armani was an under-exploited asset. He is one of the world's most famous fashion designers with a classic, understated style that is just right for the '90s."[60] The more practical reason for the designer's selection was the fact that L'Oreal owned the Armani fragrance license, which it acquired in 1989 as part of the takeover of Helena Rubenstein Cosmetics.

- In tune with the value consciousness of the '90s, Gio's starting price point began at only $40 (making it one of the lower priced prestige fragrances). L'Oreal then put in the appropriate marketing muscle—approximately $50 million over a two year launch period. L'Oreal's marketing attitude was the right one: **"L'Oreal planned to spend more the first two years than it expected to make in sales."**[61]

CHANEL AND TOMMY GIRL

The marriage of fashion and fragrance is the essence of the greatest success story in women's fragrances—Chanel No. 5. Chanel was the first designer house to "exploit the happy and profitable symbiosis between fashion and perfume."[62]

Gabrielle Chanel launched Chanel No. 5 in 1921. Chanel No. 5 was revolutionary for its day. It was the first legitimate "perfume" to come from professional perfumers. Chanel No. 5 was a new type of fragrance that was both subtle and mysterious (it used a small amount of formaldehyde to make the fragrance stable). Prior to Chanel most of the scents of the day were heavy floral scents that tended to "overpower the room."[63] Even at this early juncture, it appeared that the key to success was basically an R&D effort.

The marketing of Chanel, however, was pure genius. **The bottle was simple and giving it a number made it memorable—different yet easy to remember.** Overnight Chanel No. 5 gave the old floral scents and their elaborate containers "the dishonoring stigma of the outmoded."[64]

The marriage of fashion and fragrance still presents a potent means for developing a positioning. In late 1996, Tommy Hilfiger brought forward Tommy Girl. This entry coincided with Hilfiger's early 1996 launch into women's fashion.

A Case Study

CK ONE

The 1994 introduction of CK one represented a whole new concept in fragrance marketing. "It's not about unisex or androgyny or anything else that neutralizes you as a man or a woman. It's about being one with yourself and everyone else."[65]

Despite the revolutionary nature of the CK one fragrance, the marketing program was classic. The selection of the target market was a rifle shot—Generation Xers. The packaging was "pure" '90s—a simple aluminum and glass bottle in one hundred percent plain recycled packaging. Also in sync with the value-conscious '90s was the price point—at $25 CK one was at the lowest price tier of prestige fragrances. This price point **screamed** affordable luxury—a concept that has been fruitful across all categories throughout the 1990s. In terms of the scent itself, it has "a light, fresh, floral aroma and (with) its utilitarian look will undoubtedly appeal to men, while its caring/sharing message wins over women. It's for people who are so secure, they can share anything."[66] Backing up the program was a marketing budget in excess of $20 million the first year.

Chapter 10

HOW TO BRING A NEW WOMEN'S FACIAL MOISTURIZER TO MARKET

EARLIER WE DISCUSSED THE DIFFICULTY of getting a concept (a.k.a. "The Big Idea") to the introductory market stage. We also acknowledged the abysmal "hit rate" of new products. **New products fail because companies do not have a formal, ongoing process for concept and product evaluation.**

The next four chapters will discuss the "how-to's" for implementing a process for developing and evaluating new products. We will follow a hypothetical new facial moisturizer called DermaSmooth from concept development to market introduction.

In developing DermaSmooth, there are four checkpoints that require go/no go decisions: Preliminary Concept Development, Advertising Development, Product/Package Development, and Market Introduction. Each of these will constitute a chapter. The schematic on the next page outlines the process.

NEW PRODUCT DEVELOPMENT PROCESS			
PHASE I (CHAPTER 10)	PHASE II (CHAPTER 11)	PHASE III (CHAPTER 12)	PHASE IV (CHAPTER 13)
Preliminary Concept	Advertising Development	Product/Package	Market Introduction
Selecting	Communicating "The Big Idea"	Consumer Expectations Met	Advertising & Promotion Level
Preliminary Business Evaluation	Detailed Business Evaluation	Detailed Business Evaluation	Market Evaluations

PHASE I: PRELIMINARY CONCEPT DEVELOPMENT

The first criteria for success in developing a new beauty product is to have a **Big Idea**. This idea is usually developed through a team approach:

- **Marketing:** responsible for isolating the product category to enter.
- **Advertising Agency:** responsible for actually writing and dimensionalizing the concept (words, pictures, sound, color, etc.).
- **Research and Development:** provides a go/no go response to the agency's concept in terms of feasibility. If yes, R&D details the time frame.
- **Marketing Research:** specifies the plan for evaluating the concept, product, and advertising claims.

Thus, the starting point for a new product is the concept (a.k.a. The Big Idea). When an idea is expressed in "consumer language," it is called a concept. **If the consumer does not react positively to the concept, it is time to go back to the drawing board.** A concept is a short statement about the product. The requirements for a concept are:

- **Must** contain the product's name.
- **Must** provide both an emotional and functional benefit.
- **Must** provide a consumer-based "reason why" to believe.
- **Must** be associated with a credible "source authority."
- **Must** have a focused target group.
- **Must** contain a retail price.
- **Must** tell where the product would be available.

DERMASMOOTH'S CONCEPT

The "white care" concept (an idea presented without even a depiction of the product) for our hypothetical facial moisturizer product called DermaSmooth is as follows:

DermaSmooth helps your skin stay younger looking longer. As your skin ages, it slowly loses its ability to produce enough natural moisture. This leads to dry skin and premature wrinkles. The labs of DermaSmooth have developed an exclusive combination of moisturizing ingredients called DMS that matches your skin's own natural moisturizers. They are contained in thousands of micro moisture beads that penetrate through your skin's outer epidermis to deliver effective and natural moisture to where it is most needed. This product has been tested by leading dermatologists for more than five years and was found to provide smoother skin in less than three weeks to ninety-eight percent of the more than 20,000 test respondents. The product retails for $4.99 and is available at leading food stores, drug stores, and mass merchandiser stores.

In reading the DermaSmooth description, it is important to note that the above statement meets all the requirements for depicting a concept:

- **The product's name.** DermaSmooth—a name that conveys the fact that the product is competing in the skin care category.

- **An emotional end benefit.** DermaSmooth's emotional hook is clearly the promise of "younger looking skin."
- **A rational end benefit.** "Smoother skin in less than three weeks" is DermaSmooth's rational claim.
- **A product "reason why" to believe.** "DMS micro moisture beads" is the scientific "proof" for why the product will work.
- **A source of authority.** The recommendation by dermatologists is DermaSmooth's professional endorsement.
- **A target description.** DermaSmooth is positioned at women who want to fight the "aging process."
- **A retail price.** DermaSmooth will be sold at a suggested retail price of $4.99.
- **Product availability.** DermaSmooth's concept clearly states that it is available at leading food stores, drug stores, and mass merchandisers.

CONCEPT EVALUATION

A preliminary concept evaluation generally is conducted among an initial sample of one hundred target consumers. In the DermaSmooth example, the target consumer is a user of facial moisturizers who purchases this product in either a food store, drug store, or mass merchandiser. These target consumers customarily see only a brief written description of the idea (the DermaSmooth concept statement on the previous page).

This first screening of the idea generally does not have a picture of the product or any other imagery. The goal is to have the words conjure up an image and have each consumer react to that image. Later on when the "consumer image" is better understood, then the agency can begin the task of developing the stimuli to enhance the concept.

These consumers are asked to evaluate the idea based on a series of questions which always include: purchase interest (at a given price point), "reasons why" for purchase interest, likes/dislikes about the concept, uniqueness, believability, comparison to current brand used most often, and demographics.

Most companies have a historical "norm" that they have derived on a category and/or brand basis which states what level of purchase interest must be achieved for a preliminary concept to proceed to the next stage. Most purchase interest scales are either four point (Definitely Would Buy, Probably Would Buy, Probably Would Not Buy, or Definitely Would Not Buy) or five point scales (on these there is a middle point: Might or Might Not Buy).

Many companies still use the top two responses in setting their purchase interest goal (Definitely Would Buy and Probably Would Buy). In my experience this tends to overstate the business proposition. **The only valid purchase interest number that should drive the decision to either go forward, nix the idea totally, or revise the concept is the "Top Box" score (Definitely Would Buy).**

When the Definitely Would Buy purchase interest number is factored for awareness (how many consumers at the end of the first year heard about DermaSmooth) and distribution (the percentage of stores, weighted for their sales importance, that carried DermaSmooth) a close approximation of the first year trial can be developed.

In the case of DermaSmooth, let's assume that it achieved a 25% Definite Purchase Interest Score in the concept test. This number is then plugged into a hypothetical *Trial & Repeat model* to assess potential volume for the first year.

THE TRIAL & REPEAT MODEL

A Trial & Repeat model is a basic blueprint for assessing how likely your business proposition is to make money. This is one of

TRIAL & REPEAT MODEL

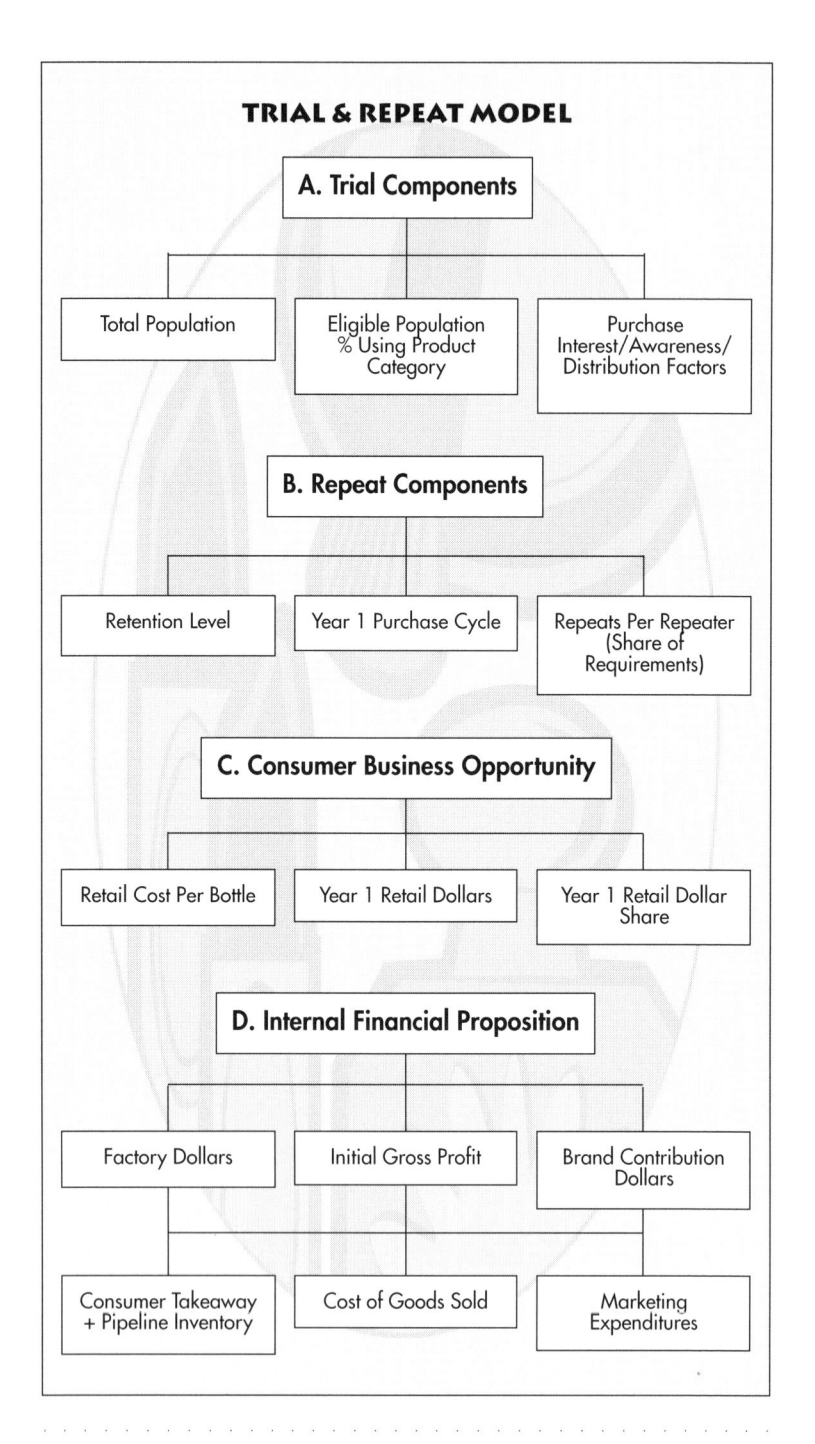

A. Trial Components

- Total Population
- Eligible Population % Using Product Category
- Purchase Interest/Awareness/Distribution Factors

B. Repeat Components

- Retention Level
- Year 1 Purchase Cycle
- Repeats Per Repeater (Share of Requirements)

C. Consumer Business Opportunity

- Retail Cost Per Bottle
- Year 1 Retail Dollars
- Year 1 Retail Dollar Share

D. Internal Financial Proposition

- Factory Dollars
- Initial Gross Profit
- Brand Contribution Dollars
- Consumer Takeaway + Pipeline Inventory
- Cost of Goods Sold
- Marketing Expenditures

the most important exercises that products go through at the preliminary concept stage and later on at the final product decision stage. It not only takes into consideration virtually all the major marketing and production expenditures, but it also incorporates into this "bottom line" the full potential of the consumer proposition. The Trial & Repeat model is composed of four primary components:

- Trial Components
- Repeat Components
- Consumer Opportunity
- Internal Financial Opportunity

TRIAL COMPONENTS

- **Eligible Population Base:** This is the percentage of consumers who are using a particular product category. In the case of facial moisturizers, it is based on the percentage of women aged 18-59 who use a facial moisturizer. The number of facial moisturizer users is derived by multiplying the female population aged 18-59 by the percentage of women that regularly use a facial moisturizer (80 million women x 65% usage level).

    A category's incidence of use level (the percentage of women that use a facial moisturizer) can be obtained through Simmons syndicated diary data. This is a data source that is available to almost every advertising agency.

    An additional source for assessing category usage is through the concept research that is being done for the preliminary concept evaluation phase. All it requires is to divide the total number of women contacted for the study by those that actually said they were regular users of a facial moisturizer product.

- **Purchase Interest—Definitely Would Buy Score (DWB):** This is the percentage of eligible target consumers who said they would buy this concept idea at the price stated if it were available at the store where they regularly purchase facial moisturizers. Assuming that DermaSmooth has obtained a 25% Definitely Would Buy Level, this equates to approximately 13 million women that would "definitely" buy this product if they saw it (52 million moisturizer users x 25% DermaSmooth DWB score).

- **Awareness:** This number is multiplied against the DWB score. It assumes that at the end of the first year a certain number of target consumers would be made aware that this product exists. My experience has been that a product that is going to compete in a competitive category, such as face care, must allocate enough marketing budget to generate at least 30% awareness in the first year.

  To accomplish this, it usually requires spending even more (on a relative basis) than the category leader in the first year in both advertising dollars and promotional expenditures (See Internal Financial Proposition in this chapter). Thus, for purposes of this example we will assume that the marketing spending plan will yield a 30% Year I awareness level for DermaSmooth.

- **Distribution:** The fact is that few products secure 100% distribution in the first year. Information Resources, Inc. classifies any product that can secure more than 50% distribution in the first year as doing extremely well. Therefore, I have assumed a 50% distribution level for DermaSmooth.

- **Total Trial Level:** This is derived by multiplying the Eligible Population (52 million) x DWB Score (25%) x Awareness Level (30%) x Distribution Level (50%). In the case of DermaSmooth, the total trial level would be 2 million women (approximately a 4% incidence level against the eligible population base: 2 million women who will try DermaSmooth divided by 52 million moisturizer users).

REPEAT COMPONENTS

- **Retention Level:** This relates to the likelihood of a onetime trier becoming a "regular" brand user. Experience dictates that a first time repeat level for a personal care product considered to be "good" by the consumer is 50%; second time repeat level is 85% of first repeaters; third time repeat level is 90% of second repeaters. After three repeat cycles, the consumer is considered a loyal user of the brand. For DermaSmooth, I have assumed that the initial retention level is 38% (50% First Time Repeat x 85% Second Time Repeat x 90% Third Time Repeat).
- **Year 1 Purchase Cycle:** During this preliminary phase, the rule of thumb is to assume that the average purchase cycle for the category also would hold true for the new product. Therefore, DermaSmooth would have a maximum of four purchases a year. Four is the average number of purchases that a facial moisturizer user makes in a year.
- **Repeats Per Repeater/Share of Requirements:** Repeats Per Repeater is the number of times that each trier will purchase the product in the first year. A "most often user" of a brand gives approximately 65-75% of her share of requirements (the total number of units purchased of any one brand divided by the total number of category purchases) to that brand. In our example, DermaSmooth will get, on average, approximately 2.5 purchases from repeaters (approximately 65% of their total facial moisturizer purchases: 2.5 DermaSmooth purchases divided by 4 facial moisturizer purchases).
- **Total Repeat Units From Triers:** This is obtained by multiplying the Trial Level x Retention Level x Repeats Per Repeater. For DermaSmooth, the total repeat level equates to 1,900,000 (2,000,000 Triers x 38% Retention Level x 2.5 Purchases).

It should be noted that a critical assumption made in our example is that each time a woman purchases DermaSmooth she buys only one unit at a time. Therefore, units and triers become one and the same number. It has been my experience that rarely is more than one product purchased at any given purchase occasion. This is especially true for a product that has a retail price point of more than $4.00 in the mass class of trade.

YEAR 1 CONSUMER BUSINESS OPPORTUNITY

- **Total Units Sold:** This is obtained by adding the Total Trial Level to the Total Repeat Level. Thus, DermaSmooth is projected to sell 3,900,000 units in Year 1 (Trial Units: 2,000,000 + Repeat Units: 1,900,000).
- **Consumer Takeaway & Retail Inventory:** Year 1 in "marketing time" usually encompasses ten months of actual consumer sales and two months of inventory (either on the retailer's shelf or in the retailer's warehouse). In other words, approximately 20% of the units that are produced will remain in inventory (either on the shelf or at the retailer's storage facilities). This has tremendous cost implications when figuring out a Year 1 business proposition. Again, a quick rule of thumb says that if the Year 1 business plan is based on twelve months, you should assume that approximately 75-80% of the units sold will be at retail prices (commonly referred to as consumer takeaway) while 20-25% will always remain in inventory (this generally is referred to as Year 1 Pipeline Inventory). DermaSmooth's consumer takeaway will be 3,120,000 (3,900,000 Total DermaSmooth Units x 80%). The balance of the 780,000 units is Pipeline Inventory.
- **Year 1 Total Retail Dollars:** This is obtained by multiplying the Effective Retail Price x Total Consumer Takeaway (it does not take into consideration the inventory component). The Effective Retail Price is the best "guesstimate" of what the

average shelf price is to the consumer. It takes into account the early introductory promotions, as well as the likely ongoing discount that retailers would give the product. It is assumed that DermaSmooth's actual retail shelf price for Year 1 would be in the neighborhood of $3.75 (the suggested retail price of $4.99 less a 25% promotional reduction). See Internal Financial Section for details.

- **Total Retail Dollar Share:** This is obtained by dividing the Total Facial Moisturizer Category Dollars by the retail dollars (consumer takeaway) expected in Year 1.

  Total category dollars for a product sold in the food, drug, or mass class of trade usually is obtained from outside vendors. The principal outside vendors who sell sales information are Information Resources, Inc., Chicago; A.C. Nielsen Co., Chicago; and Find, SVP, New York.

THE INTERNAL FINANCIAL PROPOSITION

- **Total Factory Dollars:** This is derived by multiplying Total Units Sold in Year 1 x Wholesale Price. The wholesale price is a mark down to the retailer from the suggested retail price (SRP). For beauty care products, this usually is in the range of 35-50%. DermaSmooth is assumed to have a 40% retailer margin or $3.00 wholesale price point. To derive DermaSmooth's total factory dollar volume potential in Year 1, multiply the brand's total units (3,900,000) times the wholesale price ($3.00). This yields a total of $11,700,000.

  It is important to note that this calculation includes the inventory component (both at the shelf and in the retailer's warehouse). **Pipeline Inventory is a onetime benefit that is accrued to the manufacturer.**

  Many marketers have put forth mediocre business propositions for the expressed purpose of getting the onetime benefit of Pipeline Inventory. It is a trap which can come back to haunt the manufacturer—in the form of returns. If the new product does not meet sales expectations, it is a certainty that the manufacturer will be taking back the product.

- **Cost Of Goods Sold (COG):** At the preliminary concept stage this is a "best guess" that usually is derived from historical norms. Generally, it is in the neighborhood of about 40-50% of factory sales for beauty care products. DermaSmooth's COG is estimated at 45%. This equates to a COG dollar level of $5,265,000 (Total DermaSmooth Factory Dollars of $11,700,000 x 45%).

- **Initial Gross Profit (IGP):** This is the difference between Factory Dollars and Cost Of Goods Sold. A Year 1 IGP level of 50% is considered excellent. Usually manufacturing efficiencies can bring IGP levels up three to five points over the next two or three years. The initial IGP dollars for DermaSmooth is $6,435,000 or 55% (Total DermaSmooth Factory Dollars of $11,700,000 less $5,265,000 COG).

- **Marketing Expenditures:** These include trade promotion, consumer promotion, and advertising support levels.

- **Trade Promotion:** This is usually in the neighborhood of a 25-30% level for the first year. In the following years, it tends to moderate downward to 12-15% of sales. The assumed level for DermaSmooth will be 30% in the first year or $3,510,000 (Total DermaSmooth Factory Dollars of $11,700,00 x 20%).

- **Consumer Promotion:** This is usually in the neighborhood of 20% for the first year; and then levels off to 8-15% in the "out years." The assumed level for DermaSmooth will be 20% in the first year or $2,340,000 (Total DermaSmooth Factory Dollars of $11,700,00 x 20%).

- **Advertising Levels:** This usually is derived by taking the category advertising to sales ratio (A/S) and "doubling" the level to determine a minimum advertising support level. In the mass market facial moisturizer category, the average A/S is approximately 6%. Therefore, in the hypothetical Derma-Smooth example, this would equate to a level of 12% or $1,404,000 (Total DermaSmooth Factory Dollars of $11,700,00 x 12%). In terms of the share of voice (SOV is the amount of a brand's advertising dollars divided by the advertising expenditures for the total category), this equates to approximately a three share of voice for DermaSmooth. Since its share of market is slightly less than two, this appears to be an adequate level in the first year to meet the expected volume projections. **Wrong!**

CAUTION

It should be noted that although the numbers "work" for advertising in terms of the A/S ratio and the SOV, the absolute allocation of $1.4 million is not enough to generate the required 30% brand awareness level. A consensus of knowledgeable advertising and marketing professionals believes this type of advertising expenditure is not enough to break through clutter. (See Chapter 11 for a detailed discussion of the advertising component.)

Another rule of thumb is that it requires at least a $3 million campaign today in print and a minimum $8–10 million TV advertising expenditure to get the required **reach** *(75% of the target market) and* **frequency** *(reaching that target four times in the course of a one year period) to yield 30% Year 1 brand awareness.*

It should be recognized that it will take a television campaign significantly less time than a print campaign to generate awareness; however, print is a better medium for delivering a beauty product despite the fact that it is a longer build. It has been my experience that women need to "study" beauty ads before they commit to a new product. This is especially true for a facial moisturizer. Hence, print not only gives them a longer time to review the message, but it delivers it far more personally.

- **Brand Contribution:** This is the level of IGP less marketing expenditures. DermaSmooth's Year 1 brand contribution equals a loss of $660,000.

SUMMARY

The loss for DermaSmooth in the first year is the norm for most new beauty care products today. The fact that DermaSmooth comes close to break-even says that this is an idea that has merit and should be continued. Therefore, DermaSmooth heads for the next stage: product development and advertising development.

Chapter 11

PHASE II: ADVERTISING AND PRODUCT DEVELOPMENT PROCESS

THE COPY STRATEGY

IN DEVELOPING ADVERTISING, the primary vehicle used to establish the "ground rules" is the Copy Strategy Plan. This vehicle details the Primary Target Market, Principal Benefit, Reason Why, and Tone that the advertising should take.

In the case of DermaSmooth, the Copy Strategy Document might read as follows:

PRIMARY TARGET MARKET

Women between the ages of 30–54 who are concerned about the aging process is the primary target market. They will most likely be heavy users of facial moisturizers and believers in the fact that skin care products can "slow" the effects of aging.

PRINCIPAL BENEFIT

The principal benefit of DermaSmooth is to convince women that regular use of DermaSmooth will help their skin stay younger looking and be healthier.

REASON WHY

Through DermaSmooth's exclusive combination of moisturizing ingredients called DMS, it actually can replace the moisture loss that occurs during the natural aging process.

A secondary "reason why" in terms of effective proof are the remarkable test results that have been conducted over a five-year period with thousands of respondents. Ninety-eight percent of the women tested showed significant improvement. These results are available upon request.

TONE AND MANNER

The personality of the brand will be serious in nature. It must have a scientific authenticity associated with it. However, the payoff (younger looking skin) must be demonstrated in a manner that makes the women using DermaSmooth appear confident, smart, attractive, and real.

THE DEVELOPMENT OF ADVERTISING

DETERMINING APPROPRIATE FREQUENCY & REACH LEVELS

This discussion deals with two primary elements—reach and frequency—which, in today's world, are almost dictated by the size of the budget. Since we have previously stated that

DermaSmooth will have only $3 million to spend in advertising dollars, the goal then is to create as much awareness as possible on a limited budget—this means choosing the frequency route.

Choosing frequency as the strategic operative (versus reach) means communicating to a narrower target market on a more frequent basis. In the case of DermaSmooth, we will target heavy facial moisturizer users at least three times a month over a one-year period.

THE COMPONENTS OF STRONG ADVERTISING

In developing advertising, three critical components must be assessed before giving the "go ahead" to produce final advertising. An effective commercial execution (whether it be television or print) must have the ability to register recall, communicate the main benefit (or the "reason why), and be persuasive.

- **Recall** is the first hurdle that advertising must overcome. If consumers can't remember a message, they won't be persuaded to buy it. Recall of an advertising execution must be viewed in a competitive environment—a *broad* competitive environment. My definition of competition today is the total of all advertising done in the same medium. Therefore, **the ability of any advertising to break through the sea of ads available on television or in magazines must be the first barrier that an effective ad must overcome.** This element is commonly referred to as "breaking through clutter." DermaSmooth's principal competitive frame will be all other beauty or personal care products—a formidable task indeed.
- **Communication** is the second hurdle. This refers to the advertising's ability to get its main point across. The key here is to make sure that the communication is such that it **establishes a clear point of difference between the new product and competition.** In the case of DermaSmooth, the

DMS micro moisture beads should be the "reason why" this product can work better than traditional facial moisturizers.
- **Persuasion** is the third and the most important characteristic that an effective advertising execution must have. **Persuasion is the ultimate payoff.** As stated previously, the only valid indication of this element is the "definitely would buy score." **If this score does not generate a level that is significantly greater than that obtained in the "white card" preliminary concept phase (25% in the DermaSmooth example) then the advertising should not go forward.** By holding to this ideal, it ensures that advertising has, in fact, made the proposition even more inviting by bringing it to life both verbally and visually.

SELECTING THE ADVERTISING MEDIUM

In deciding on the advertising medium, the general consensus among advertising agency executives is that television advertising should not be conducted with less than an $8–10 million working media budget. Working media refers to the actual number of impressions that the consumer will see (working media does not include the costs of producing or testing the advertising). Since DermaSmooth will have an advertising budget of $3 million, the medium of choice should be print advertising.

I must emphasize, however, that even if the budget were such that television could be a consideration, **I fully believe that the real test of an agency's ability to communicate a positioning should be done first as a print execution (i.e. a "billboard" approach). If a two-dimensional medium can accurately translate a positioning, then the chances of a successful television execution is enhanced enormously.**

MELDING FUNCTIONAL AND EMOTIONAL ELEMENTS TOGETHER

Regardless of the medium used to develop the execution, the end goal is to effectively fuse together the functional (the mind) and emotional (the heart) elements. (See the chart in Chapter 1). In the DermaSmooth example, creating an emotional attachment to the viewer is critical (looking younger is by definition an emotional message). Further, there is significant evidence that, when advertising can trigger an emotional arousal, overall communication of product benefits are enhanced.[1]

In the mid-1980s, David Zeitlin and Richard Westwood of the Beaumont Organization, a strategic research company in Tarrytown, New York, found in their research that emotion can be directly linked to three separate and distinct elements of communication:

- **Emotions can be benefits.** Emotions can play a fundamental role in the purchase of a product or category. In the case of DermaSmooth, the emotional concept of "looking younger" evokes one of the most powerful emotions in beauty care marketing.
- **Emotions can communicate benefits.** An emotional tone can draw attention to a message, making it extremely memorable. An example of this is the allegorical Lubriderm alligator, which implies "rough skin."
- **Emotions can directly influence attitudes.** Extensive and appropriate theme advertising appears to imbue some brands with a subjective vividness, a glamour, or an authenticity that comparable competitors lack[2]. In these cases, the brand name is consistently presented in conjunction with the evocation of an emotion and, in time, comes to evoke the emotion itself. **Preference by L'Oreal with its signature theme, "I'm worth**

it," is an example of how an emotional response can directly influence an attitude.

ADVERTISING TESTING SERVICE COMPANIES

In developing the print campaign for DermaSmooth, the advertising agency generally will try a number of different pictorial layouts. Each of these different executions should be tested to ensure that recall, communication, and persuasion levels have been met. There are a number of companies that test print executions. In my experience, however, I have found that Video Storyboards is one of the best. It provides "normative" levels for each of the above measures and, more importantly, insight as to what works and what needs improvement. Video Storyboards is located in New York City.

Chapter 12:
PHASE III: PACKAGING AND PRODUCT DEVELOPMENT

PACKAGE DEVELOPMENT
THE PACKAGE DESIGN AND GRAPHICS have a much stronger and longer term impact on sales than either advertising or promotion. Over the long haul, this is what the consumer sees on a day in/day out basis. It is the embodiment of the brand's personality. **It must be able to attract, engage, inform, and motivate the shopper—all in a matter of seconds.**[3]

THE PACKAGING BRIEF
The package development process is much like that for advertising; it starts with the Packaging Brief. The Packaging Brief is the basic document that details the strategy and objectives of the packaging. Continuing with our hypothetical DermaSmooth example, the

following might be representative of the main objectives that would be detailed in DermaSmooth's Packaging Brief:

- It must reinforce the brand's positioning as the product that will make women look younger—and so, help them look and feel their confident best every day.
- It must maximize shelf impact and registration, while strongly communicating the DermaSmooth name. Additionally, and most importantly, it must differentiate itself from other competition.
- The package must lend itself to periodic line extensions (such as, a product for sensitive skin). In this regard, thought must be given to how to differentiate sub-brands/types within the line while maintaining line compatibility.
- Packaging must allow for periodic announcements of special consumer offers on the front label in an intrusive, yet image sensitive manner.

THE PACKAGING TESTING PROCESS

Since the product's shelf presence is the only marketing force in constant touch with the consumer, it is even more important that this element be assessed to ensure that the above objectives are being met. In the case of package testing, the process is similar to advertising testing; however, there are some variations.

In advertising testing, I noted that the first hurdle rate was recall; in package testing, this is called visibility (the ability to find the product on the shelf). Visibility is akin to "breaking through clutter," where clutter refers to the "sea of shelf competition." Visibility is sometimes referred to as "shopability." The key in this phase is to assess how long it takes the average category shopper to find the product on the shelf.

The second hurdle rate identified in advertising testing was communication; this is the same issue for package testing. The packaging should communicate the same message as the advertising in terms of the positioning. The DermaSmooth packaging and graphics must be able to communicate that it is a product that will help women look younger.

The "purchase interest" commitment noted for advertising is also critical in package development. However, because there are certain fixed parameters for packaging in categories that are already well established, there generally is less noticeable innovation in design. Therefore, much of the onus for the "definite purchase interest" level is put squarely on the shoulders of the graphics.

PRODUCT DEVELOPMENT

For the most part, the new products development process is today a shared vision. In days gone by it was principally engineered by marketing. Marketing would give its concept statement to research and development, and R&D would be expected to make the concept a reality. However, with product proliferation being rampant and the number of new items being introduced at quicker time intervals (such as 10,000-15,000 new items each year), the chances for success also have gotten correspondingly slimmer (See Chapter 2).

DEVELOPING A PRODUCT: THE PROCESS

Therefore, most sophisticated beauty care companies have turned to R&D as a full partner in the concept development process. As noted early, R&D is a member of the new products team from the inception of the idea up until final introduction into the marketplace. **During the concept development stage, R&D should be challenged with thinking about specific product properties: texture, application techniques, line extensions or shade extensions (as in the case of color cosmetics), and cost and timing limitations.**[4]

This information is developed through extensive communication between marketing and R&D.[5] This step is critical in determining a product's feasibility and often fine tunes the original product profile.[6]

R&D "MUST HAVES": CRITICAL ELEMENTS OF SUCCESS

It should be noted that for product development to be successful, it requires that marketing spend a lot of time with R&D to ensure that this group understands the concept. The key is that the product deliver on its stated promise to the specific target market. In the case of DermaSmooth, the critical target is 30+ and the goal is to actually have the product make its users look younger. Colgate-Palmolive has an excellent single-minded focus in terms of how it views the development of a specific product. Colgate's development premise starts and ends with the following belief: *"our goal is to ensure that our products delight potential target consumers."*

The concept of "delight" is a statement that embodies more than just quality; it requires an intense focus on creativity and actual product delivery.[7]

This section would not be complete without at least a mention of the influence that the global marketplace has on product and concept development. Most products introduced today are made with the thought that they will have (or at least should have) international potential. To truly benefit from the international environment, however, marketers and R&D folks alike must be attuned to the differences in consumer behavior between countries and regions. Again utilizing the DermaSmooth example, although the desire for "younger looking skin" is a motivating benefit regardless of international boundary, how you deliver that benefit matters significantly. For example, a cream formulation may be desirable in the United States, but lotions rule in Latin America, and oils in the Far East.

BLIND PRODUCT TESTING VERSUS IDENTIFIED PRODUCT TESTING

Once the product is developed, the next phase is to ensure that it, in fact, delivers on the concept promise (that it delights the consumer). Thus, management now needs to assess if the DermaSmooth promise of "younger looking skin" is delivered. This testing process usually is conducted via a twofold procedure.

The first phase is commonly referred to as a *blind product test*.

BLIND PRODUCT TESTING

A blind product test usually is conducted between the new formulation and either the current category leader and/or the leader in the particular segment of a category that the new product is targeted against. DermaSmooth is clearly being positioned as a facial moisturizer targeted to women 30+. Therefore, it should be tested against the leading mass facial moisturizer: Oil of Olay. Additionally, because there is significant competition in this market, I also would test DermaSmooth against the other formidable competitor, Ponds Facial Cream (Ponds also has an older skew, thereby, further justifying its need for testing). Lastly, because the promise of younger looking skin is clearly going against Revlon's successful Age Defying Facial Moisturizer entry, this too should be assessed.

In this hypothetical blind product test, four panels of consumers will be matched on the basis of their frequency and brand usage of facial moisturizers. Each person will be given one of the products to try, but she will not know which brand she is using. The products will be given to each consumer in a white, opaque jar that will have only the R&D number on it. Thus, one panel will be given DermaSmooth, the second panel Oil of Olay, the third panel Ponds, and the fourth panel Revlon's Age Defying Facial Moisturizer.

Each consumer will use the product for a two-week period. They will use the product as they would their normal facial moisturizer brand. At the end of the two-week period, they will be contacted and questioned regarding product likes, dislikes, purchase interest, and specific attributes. The key will be to assess how the DermaSmooth formulation matches up to its potential competition.

THE CONCEPT/PRODUCT TEST

I believe that this is the most important part of any testing process. It is the embodiment of all the work that has been put forward. In this phase, the company repeats the concept test, but this time using finished advertising (in the case of DermaSmooth, the recommended introductory print ad). Thus, after exposure to the print ad ("please read this ad and then we will ask you some questions about it") respondents are again queried regarding likes, dislikes, purchase interest, product attribute ratings, psychographic characteristics, uniqueness, and believability. After the concept phase, the respondents in the study are asked to try DermaSmooth for a two-week period. Here, the same questions obtained in the blind product testing phase and in the concept phase are asked again. The difference, however, is that in this phase of the testing process we are exposing final packaging and formulation. Again, utilizing a product usage period of two weeks is fairly standard procedure.

The key is to then match the concept delivery with the product delivery. Did DermaSmooth deliver on its consumer promise of "younger looking skin"?

SUMMARY

When the concept results and product results are received these levels are then used to update the Trial & Repeat model that was developed. **This serves as a significant refinement of the business proposition.**

Chapter 13:

PHASE IV: MARKET INTRODUCTION

INTRODUCTORY TRADE PROMOTION LEVEL

ONE REASON THAT I CHOSE THE FACIAL moisturizer category for the introduction of a new product (our DermaSmooth example) is that it is a beauty care segment that has been in a state of constant transition over the past few years. Moisturizer brands (whether they be line extensions or new products) have been introduced at an ever increasing rate (this is consistent with the growth in the 35+ population).

The constant flow of new products is due to the nature of the beauty care industry. It plays on consumers' wishes to find the ultimate "hope in a jar"; in fact, the promise of youth is so compelling that the newest "new news" generally receives some level of attention.

However, the truth is that category leaders such as Olay, Ponds, and Revlon still remain one, two, and three in brand share levels.[8] Obviously, this speaks to the high loyalty level of this category and the fear that users have that an unknown entity will cause a physical condition (such as an allergic reaction) or, perhaps more importantly, emotional stress from that potentially negative physical reaction.

As stated in Chapter 4, the average sales promotion spending rate for an established beauty care product is about 15% of net sales. However, in the case of new products, that level escalates to at least 25%. For categories that have high loyalty levels such as facial moisturizers, this can range as high as 30% in the first year.

Since the purchase cycles tend to be elongated in the facial moisturizer category (approximately one purchase every ten to twelve weeks), **it is necessary to maintain these high deal levels throughout the first year to ensure maximum consumer trial and strong trade support** (in terms of feature ads, displays, or just temporary shelf price reductions).

INTRODUCTORY CONSUMER PROMOTION LEVEL

Consumer promotion is the other key ingredient in the manufacturer's promotional arsenal. Consumer promotion can take the form of direct to consumer sampling efforts, couponing endeavors (in terms of both instant redeemable coupons as well as cents off for future purchases), sweepstakes, trial size introductions, etc.

For a new product, the level generally approaches 20% of net sales. Therefore, for our DermaSmooth example, this equates to approximately $2.5 million.

THE BALANCE BETWEEN ADVERTISING AND PROMOTION

In our DermaSmooth example, we have assumed a thirty percent trade promotion level ($4 million), a twenty percent consumer promotion level ($2.5 million), and a $3 million advertising budget. The table below depicts the relative importance (in percentage) of each of these marketing expenditures.

The relationships depicted above for advertising, consumer promotion, and trade promotion levels are in line with historical levels for personal care products.[9]

DERMASMOOTH
RELATIONSHIP OF MARKETING EXPENDITURES

Trade Promotion	42%
Consumer Promotion	26%
Advertising Expenditures	32%

THE RETAILER/MANUFACTURER RELATIONSHIP

For DermaSmooth to be successful, it requires a close tie-in between the manufacturer and the retailer. Successful retailers make the most out of their major vendor's marketing strengths.

In a June 1995 interview with *Discount Store News*, Cindy Quinn, a divisional merchandise manager of cosmetics, accessories, and jewelry at Bradlees (a major North Eastern Mass Merchandiser), described the way Bradlees and Revlon have worked together. In my view, this is the prototypical way that new products must be introduced and supported if they are to be successful: "Revlon probably does it best. When they introduced their ColorStay line last June, they took out full-page ads and pullouts in magazines like *Glamour* and *Vogue* and offered customers an instant coupon. We then promoted those items in our circulars and in pre-packs in the stores.[10]

"The instant coupon Revlon offers in magazines inspires sales. If a woman sees the ad and she comes into Bradlees for what she needs, she's likely to wander into the cosmetics department with the coupon and give the product a try."[11]

Revlon also entices women to purchase their products by giving them a "free taste"[12]. In April 1995, Revlon kicked off a spring and summer promotional campaign to better familiarize 100,000 women across the country with its ColorStay and Age Defying lines. Revlon took to the road from New York and Los Angeles in two trailers equipped with beauty consultants and free samples of Age Defying makeup and ColorStay lipstick. "Mobile marketing" has since become an effective tool that many companies are using.

In the words of Tanya Mandor, Revlon's senior vice president of color cosmetics: "We're bringing a beauty message to women where they are every day—in malls, offices, close to their homes. There's no pressure, nothing to buy or subscribe to. Just great samples and advice."[13]

These are excellent examples of how the power of promotional programs, in conjunction with advertising, can develop a business. In the case of DermaSmooth, I would follow the path of Revlon as a means of increasing the chances of success.

Chapter 14

MEN'S PERSONAL CARE MARKET

MEN ARE MORE ANXIOUS TODAY than at any other time in the past quarter century, because their traditional role of **"sole provider/breadwinner" is being dislodged.** In the 1960s and 1970s, the roles of men and women were separate and unequal (yet *clearly* defined—"Men earned the bread; women went to the store to buy it!")[1]. Today, men and women often are "equal partners" in terms of household income, and the role of men is not so clearcut. **Marketers who wish to be successful in the men's personal care market must** *provide males with "self-confident" themes.* A constant reminder and reassurance of masculinity is still the key to winning in all segments of men's toiletries.

Men in the 1990s will continue to experience "major transitions." They will move from living alone to living with a partner, to marriage, to family, and through divorce back to living alone.[2] **"Singlehood" will be a state for more than forty percent of Boomers at some point in the next two decades.**[3] As a result of living alone for longer periods of time, men will take on the management of their own households and have to deal with combining home and work responsibilities.[4] As these men form

173

families, new or otherwise, they will bring these skills with them. This pattern of changing family and living arrangements with unprecedented frequency has significant implications for men in their role as consumers of personal care products.

Even those men who stay within the traditional sphere of marriage and children will have a different attitude than those men in prior generations. They too will be much more actively involved in the household as a full partner in both the shopping and child rearing duties (because more than seventy percent of men between the ages of 25 and 44 will have working wives).[5]

As the year 2000 approaches, many more men will face the same challenges that have confronted women for the past three decades: balancing the competing demands of work and home. As consumers, men may join women in developing an interest in products and services that save time or reduce the stress of juggling these responsibilities.

Successful marketing in the male personal care market will be based on providing products that couple convenience with quality and value. "The male consumer is looking for no-nonsense, lifestyle-friendly products. He wants products that do what they say they are going to do. Success will come from those manufacturers that provide products that offer benefits that are better than competitors or that are unique. Male consumers buying grooming products are willing to pay a premium for products that will deliver."[6]

MEN'S PERSONAL CARE MARKET

The primary segments of the men's personal care market are body cleansers, deodorants, shaving products, fragrances, and hair grooming products.

WHAT DRIVES PERSONAL CARE PURCHASES BY MEN?

There are five primary drivers that will influence every product segment of the men's personal care market in the years ahead:

KEY DRIVERS

- Market dynamics
- Demographic dynamics
- Lifestyle dynamics
- Trade channel dynamics
- Influence of research and development

MARKET DYNAMICS

In 1995, the men's personal care market in the United States stood at $7.7 billion.[7] Growth, although not spectacular, has been steady at roughly four percent per year since 1990.[8] However, most prognosticators are assuming that, in the next five years, this category will almost double in size because of increased media attention, education, and the realization

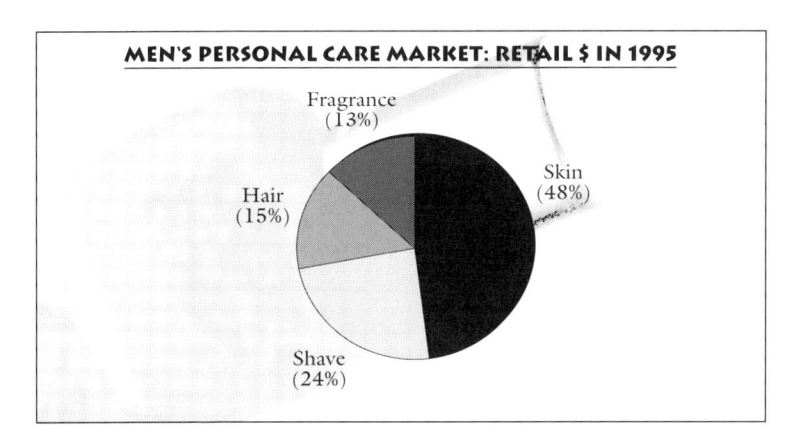

MEN'S PERSONAL CARE MARKET: RETAIL $ IN 1995

- Fragrance (13%)
- Hair (15%)
- Shave (24%)
- Skin (48%)

Source: Frost & Sullivan, U.S. Men's Personal Care Products, "Men's Personal Care Market Growing" Research Alert; September 16, 1994.

that personal care grooming regimes don't have to be complicated, expensive, or "just for women." Thus, both mass market and prestige companies are firing up their existing lines by adding new products, new fragrances, more choices, and extra benefits (including "magic ingredients" such as alpha hydroxy acids).

The male personal care market is comprised of four primary segments, with body cleansing/skin care being the largest by far.

IMPORTANCE OF DEMOGRAPHICS

Demographics rule in the marketing of men's products. Since 1980, adult males 40–59 years of age have been increasing at a clip of 2.5 percent per annum versus a less than one percent rate for adult males 20–39 years old.[9] The skew between older and younger males has gotten much closer. (In 1995, men 40-59 years old accounted for nearly forty-five percent of the total population of adult males 20–59 years of age.)[10] As a result the opportunities for segmenting products have not only become more attractive, but mandatory given the differences in needs.

The aging of the Boomers has accelerated growth in both skin care and hair care. **Growth in men's skin care has been driven by anti-aging and dual benefit products—products that both clean and moisturize—while hair care products primarily have been driven by hair coloring and hair thickening products.**

The most difficult group to market will continue to be male Xers. Just like other generations, male Xer attitudes are shaped by their experiences—and their experiences generally have not been positive. By and large, they are an angry group, particularly in terms of the workplace; they are entering the work force at a time of prolonged downsizing and downturn, so they're likelier than the previous generation to be unemployed, underemployed, and living at home with Mom and Dad.[11] In short, this is the generation of diminished expectations—the opposite of the "positive" Boomers who grew up thinking anything was possible.[12]

To a large extent, this group has a right to be cynical concerning the job market, personal relationships, and the American dream. Real wages fell by more than twenty-four percent from 1970 to 1993 among men 25-34 years of age (this is the only comparative data from the U.S. Bureau of Labor Statistics that comes close to this age group).[13]

Unlike the Boomers before them who grew up in the era of the "sexual revolution," Xers are growing up in the era of AIDS. Further, they generally do not have the benefit of emotional security, which the Boomers had. Boomers essentially grew up in a traditional family environment in which Dad went to work and Mom stayed home. Xers grew up with divorce (fifty percent of Xers' families experienced divorce),[14] and most households were two family wage earners (fifty-six percent).[15] The result is that **Xers have relatively little brand or product loyalty compared to prior generations.**

IMPACT OF LIFESTYLE CHANGES

Beyond demographics, lifestyle changes also have had a major impact on men's personal care products and men's receptivity to such products. Men who are doing more of the household shopping have become significantly more receptive to skin care and fragrance products. Men increasingly buy their own products, and manufacturers and retailers are altering their marketing strategies to respond to this shift.

Women also have helped push the need for skin care products among men. Women, being much more involved and, therefore, "educated" about skin care, have been imparting this information to men at an accelerated rate (whether they be wives, significant others, or "just the girl friend").[16]

In addition, changes in men's personal care tastes have brought greater use of unisex products in both skin care and fragrances (CK one again being the prime innovator of this phenomenon).

Marketers are increasingly coming to the realization that products specifically geared for gender may be unnecessary. Certainly it simplifies the message, while it also provides an added benefit to both the consumer and retailer—less clutter in the cabinet and less clutter on the store shelf.

It is an undeniable fact: The number of families that have income levels over $50,000 has increased over the past quarter century. In 1970, only twenty percent of families earned $50,000 or more; whereas by 1993 (the latest census data available for household income information), this number was approaching one-third of all families (in constant 1970 dollars).[17] In these households, nearly sixty percent of the women do not work outside the home; and, therefore, the total income in these households are dependent on the "male" wage earner. The propensity of these men to buy more upscale grooming products is significantly higher than for any other male group classification.

IMPACT OF CHANGING TRADE DYNAMICS

Throughout the past decade, the department store prestige distributed treatment products have been growing significantly faster than mass market brands. The primary reason is the presence of knowledgeable customer service salespersons (who also can provide samples) and the continued expansion of men's prestige lines as a separate entity from "the women's section."[18] In recent years, however, some of the more upscale drug chains (such as CVS) are beginning to have their own version of the "male oriented section" (which is significantly expanded from the more traditional single shelf of male grooming aids). **The real growth at the mass level will come from the large discounters (Wal-Mart, Kmart, and Target) when they truly have their own "male cosmetic sections."** Marketers need to push these retailers into being more proactive regarding male toiletries and grooming products if this is to become a reality.

INFLUENCE OF RESEARCH AND DEVELOPMENT

Technological developments have brought increased use of multipurpose shampoos and soaps (such as 3-in-1 products combining shampoo, conditioner, and shine enhancers).[19] Another growing area in men's toiletries is transparent or clear products for skin and hair care—such as clear shampoos, soaps, and deodorants[20]—which are gaining popularity because of their perceived purity.

Most of this innovation has come about because marketers are taking advantage of the technology in women's products and providing them (via different positionings and packaging) to men.[21]

Nevertheless marketers, if they are to be successful, must expand their customer base (this is especially true in the prestige segment). Thus, **the real home run is to expand the number of products men will use by making a "regimen" approach to skin care as important to men as it is currently for women.**

About ten years ago, Sue G. Phillips, then the director of marketing for Lancome Men's Line, hit the real issue when she said, "Men respond to a vocabulary they can understand and call their own, so we use masculine words like 'well-groomed,' 'good-looking skin,' and 'comfortable skin'."[22] Over the years, the primary gains in marketing men's products have tended to be in the "comfort zone" end of the vocabulary. Thus, men unlike women "...don't want to know that a product has collagen or elastin; they want to know what is going to happen and when it is going to happen..."[23]

BODY CLEANSERS

In the case of men, the vast majority of skin care usage revolves around the "shower experience." Men, more so than women, tend to be habitual and regimented in their cleansing routine.

More than ninety percent of men shower daily—half in the morning (before work) and about half at night (right before bed). It is during this time that they are using most of their skin care products (shampoos, conditioners, and deodorants). Nearly all men use both a shampoo and a bar soap in the shower; while more than a third of men also use a conditioning product (either a shampoo that contains a conditioner or a separate conditioning product). The shampoos generally used are "value" brands (such as Suave) or "treatment products" (Head & Shoulders, Selsun Blue, or Denorex).

In terms of the bar soap product, men unequivocally prefer deodorant soaps (nearly two-thirds of men are using deodorant soap).[26] Further, unlike women, men tend to use the same soap on their body as they do on their face.[27] If they are not using deodorant soap, then they are using either the "all family" brands (Lever 2000) or "value" brands (Ivory). **There is no question that the most salient positioning for a bar soap is the dual promise of "clean" and "providing deodorant protection."**

When men are finished with their shower, virtually all put on their deodorant; approximately sixty percent use a cologne or after shave; and nearly twenty-five percent use a skin moisturizer (either a hand and body lotion or facial moisturizer—usually in the form of a "shaving balm").[28]

MALE DEODORANT MARKET

A Case Study

COLGATE'S MENNEN DEODORANT: THE ART OF LAUNCHING A MALE DEODORANT PRODUCT

Mennen is by far the undisputed king of the male deodorant market. Mennen's success is clearly evidenced by the fact that nearly every major marketer of personal care products was after this jewel. The 1993 purchase of Mennen by Colgate brought

Colgate an instantaneous ten U.S. share brand and, more importantly, a worldwide launching platform. Mennen has written the rules in marketing deodorant products, and every successful entry has since followed these bylaws:

- To be successful in this segment, **you must establish yourself in terms of one form first (either a stick, roll-on, or aerosol).** A good example of a single-minded form introduction was Faberge's "Power Stick" deodorant entry in the late 1980s. Mennen owns the stick deodorant segment, while Gillette's Right Guard owns the aerosol market.[29] Once established, most brands have built their business through the introduction of new forms.
- **Cost of Entry in the category is the promise of protection from wetness and odor.** Mennen understood that, for men, focusing first on efficacy (protection from odor and wetness) was a lot more single-minded and, therefore, persuasive than adding a "social confidence" measure.
- Mennen also understood that to be successful, **this category requires continued advertising pressure**. Historically, Mennen's share of advertising dollars ("share of voice") has been higher than its market share.[30] This speaks to the fact that this category is a long-term build and requires patience to develop (as a function of the high loyalty levels toward deodorant brands).
- In developing a successful platform, Mennen, Power Stick, Brut, and Old Spice have all demonstrated the **need to establish one-on-one intimacy with the viewer.** Further, all the successful commercial executions rely on only one form; no brand relies on one execution to sell all forms—stick, roll-on, or aerosol.

MEN'S SHAVING PRODUCTS

Gillette controls two-thirds of the $1.3 billion men's razor and blade shaving market. Ever since the 1990 introduction of the Sensor Razor followed by the 1994 introduction of the Sensor Exel, this category has been propelled by new product introductions. At eleven percent growth, it was the third fastest growing segment of any personal care or beauty product in 1995 (behind women's and men's hair coloring products).[32] In addition, Gillette controls twenty-five percent of the shave cream dollar market (only one share point below the category leader, S. C. Johnson's Edge).[33]

Case Study
GILLETTE'S SENSOR FOR WOMEN
Successfully Piggybacking Technology To Launch Gender Specific Products. *Gillette also has taken a page from successful cosmetic manufacturers (those who have leveraged their women's skin care expertise into men's products) and has used its technology to develop the "best" women's shaving products via the Sensor For Women's Razor. Between 1993 and 1995, the women's shaving category grew by thirty percent— thanks mainly to the Sensor For Women's Razor. (In 1995, the women's shaving category was nearly $350 million.)[34] The Sensor For Women brand controls approximately one-third of the total sales for this segment.[35] The good news for Gillette was that it was able to piggyback the R&D costs for the Sensor For Men in developing the Sensor For Women. Sensor For Women R&D costs were only $10 million—about five percent of the cost for developing Sensor For Men.[36]*

To understand the success of Gillette, one need only to go to its mission statement. Ron Rossi, president of Gillette North America, summarizes it best: "If there's a better way to shave, Gillette is going to find it and we're the ones who are going to develop it."[37]

Gillette's success is based on its unabiding belief in technological advances (it spent nearly $200 million in R&D to develop the Sensor Razor for Men) and its commitment to marry such advances to significant marketing support levels. Again, Rossi succinctly captures Gillette's philosophy: "Create products that can really be differentiated and then promote the hell out of them with both consumers and the trade."[38] These words are not idle whimsy; in 1994, Gillette spent $545 million on advertising and $533 million on sales promotion.[39]

The success of this philosophy has not been lost on Wall Street. Heather Hay, a J.P. Morgan analyst, wrote in a 1995 report, "The company has an extraordinarily strong brand name, dominant market shares, technological superiority, and global reach—qualities not often found all in one package."[40]

NEW NEWS IN SHAVING

Since every man universally desires a "better shave," there is no more powerful claim that can be made. However, to be successful, it is mandatory to have technological advances to propel this claim (as in the case for all Gillette products). Nevertheless, other new products for shaving are taking the Gillette lead in terms of "new news" when it comes to shaving. To this end, the most obvious product innovations in the late 1990s have come from manufacturers specifically designing products for the African-American male.

Approximately two-thirds of all black men suffer from "pseudofolliculitis barbae" (razor bumps), a condition in which the tightly curled hairs of the beard grow back into the skin, causing small bumps on the face that conventional razors often rip open.[41]

In early 1995, BioCosmetic Research Labs, a three-year-old company, introduced Black Opal, "the first complete collection of scientifically advanced products for the care and treatment of black skin."[42] This is a regimen type product that has a cleanser (utilizing alpha hydroxy acids), a desensitizing shaving gel (to lubricate), and an after shave relief lotion.[43] These products are similar to systems that previously were available only to women. This is yet another example of taking a product developed for one gender and positioning it for the other gender.

As the intensity level for incremental dollars increases, more and more mainstream cosmetic companies (at both the class and mass level) will be coming out with male-oriented regimen systems.

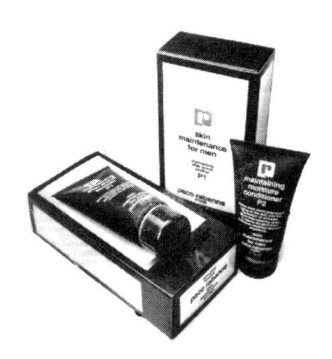

Case Study

PACO RABANNE'S SKIN MAINTENANCE FOR MEN — WHY CERTAIN PRODUCTS FAIL

A discussion of men's skin care grooming would not be complete without at least a mention of the forerunner of all male regimen skin care systems— Paco Rabanne's Skin Maintenance For Men introduced in 1984.[44]

This product nearly had all the ingredients for success— cleansers and scrubs; moisturizers and conditioners. However, it lacked the key element—the shave cream. Thus, if Paco Rabanne had developed the moisturizer as a shave cream and then surrounded it with the other products, it probably would have been a huge success. **The lesson: don't try to change behavior—improve upon it.**

MALE FRAGRANCES (COLOGNES AND AFTER SHAVES)

The male fragrance category is one of the most difficult categories to successfully market. For the most part, fifty percent of sales must be achieved in approximately a six-week window (the formidable Christmas season).[45] It also is one of the few categories that a consumer has the opportunity to try and reject prior to a purchase (nearly all products have shelf "testers"). Even more difficult from a launch positioning standpoint is the fact that roughly fifty percent of first time trial is through "gift purchases."[46] This presents another obstacle—the purchaser is not necessarily the wearer, which provides yet another opportunity for rejection by the "gift recipient."

Given the above, the most important element in successfully marketing a male fragrance product is developing a compelling product positioning and being able to demonstrate that positioning through an equally powerful visual. **In developing this positioning, the marketer must create a curiosity about the fragrance that makes the image appear "larger than life."** In developing a positioning, there are five recurring themes that appear to continue to bring forth success: sexual domination, physical strength, sincerity/belonging, attention getting, and achieving.

The fragrances Gravity and tommy both do an excellent job of utilizing two different themes to get across their positioning. Gravity relies on a combination of sexual domination and physical strength, while tommy uses sincerity/belonging to communicate its positioning. In essence, the visuals are the positioning.

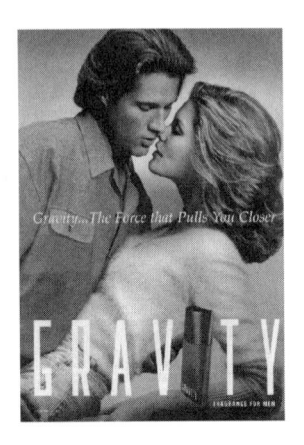

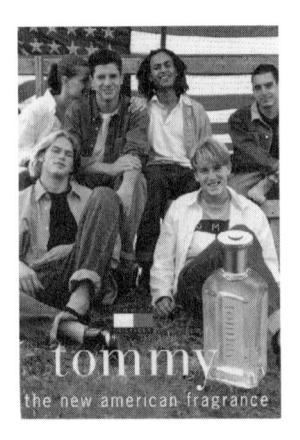

For the last few years, most of the excitement in men's fragrances have been at the designer level (tommy, Obsession, Eternity, Gravity, Polo, and Ralph Lauren).[47] However, in the 1995 Christmas season and through the second half of 1996, mass marketers began to put forth new products that take advantage of what has been going on in the prestige men's fragrance market. Several alternative designer fragrances, most notably unisex scents (ala CK one) have had some success (Parfum de Coeur's U, Delagar's Gender One, and Jean Phillippe's A Man and A Woman).[48] Coty is building on its success with its women's Vanilla Scent, by putting forth Raw Vanilla for men.[49] **Thus, successful marketing means knowing when to take a strong idea in "class" and bring it to "mass."**

A Case Study

PIERRE CARDIN: HOW TO BRING "CLASS TO MASS"

Tsumura International's Pierre Cardin fragrance has had real success since it was brought into the mass class of trade. Although this is always a sensitive area (bringing a product from "class to mass"), there are a number of instances when this can be a successful strategy. One only has to look at Revlon's success since it went to a "high end mass brand."

186 *Beauty and the Beastly Market*

The "reason why" Pierre Cardin has been successful is that the marketers at Tsumura really understood that Pierre Cardin appeals to an older "mature market" (the Baby Boomers that have graduated into the next classification). By maintaining a fairly high price point in both drug and discounters, Tsumura has been able to maintain Pierre Cardin's prestige image while making it "accessibly affordable." Importantly, Tsumura has never denigrated the brand's "preciousness" by offering significant discounts (thereby maintaining the brand's upscale identity while at the same time keeping the margins healthy).

This category thrives on continually relaunching established products. It's important to remember that for the past ten years Procter & Gamble's Old Spice, Faberge's Brut, Coty's Stetson, Jovan, and Preferred Stock have controlled more than fifty percent of the mass market share (approximately $250 million in retail dollars).[50] They have been able to accomplish this through: continually reviving brands via new line extensions (new scents like Aqua Velva's 1994 Ice Sport entry for younger men and Brut's Brut Actif Blue, a fragrance for younger males who participate in "high-energy activities"); updating packaging (sprays in addition to traditional bottles and updated graphics for old standbys as in the case of Canoe and Navy For Men); and providing constant marketing support (both at the trade promotion level and consumer level). Beyond the constant marketing fine tuning, sales of fragrances also have been positively affected by the move of some of them into the men's grooming section of the store.[51] **Hence, opportunities also can be had by paying close attention to in-store placement; micro-marketing can be a potent avenue to success.**

Another technique being used increasingly at the mass level is to generate incremental sales via extending mature fragrance brands into other product segments. To this end, J.B. Williams doubled its spending on its "aging" Aqua Velva brand to $10 million in 1996 as it introduced seven new products into this 70-year-old fragrance.[52] These new Aqua Velva products included a deodorant and antiperspirant. Thus, like Old Spice and Brut years before, Aqua Velva hopes to translate its strength as a fragrance to deodorants.

Robert Sheasby, the vice president of marketing at J.B. Williams (and formerly from Chesebrough-Ponds, the leader in skin care marketing), says, "It's a huge undeveloped area for us. The trend is toward fragrance-based brand loyalty."[53]

One of the more interesting occurrences in the 1990s was the beginning of a "value segment" in the department store class of trade. The innovator in this development was Ralph Lauren's Polo Sport's Water Basic line of skin treatment and fragrances introduced in 1995. It was priced at $15, which made it $8 less than Clinique's products and $12 less than Aramis' products.

Polo has marketed its whole line as a "fitness fragrance" and priced it affordably. Camille McDonald, the senior vice president of marketing for Ralph Lauren, explained, "Men won't pay for these products the way women will. Men tend to buy grooming products in drug stores, so we have very affordable pricing versus usual prices available at department stores."[54]

MEN'S HAIR GROOMING CATEGORY

A Case Study

COMB'S: HOW GENERATIONAL MARKETING COUPLED WITH ATTENTION TO MICRO-MARKETING ELEMENTS EQUALS SUCCESS.

Men's hair coloring products are the fastest growing segment in men's hair preparations.[55] Comb's Just For Men Hair Coloring Product (which now owns this segment with a share in excess of forty percent)[56] is a good example of generational marketing. It *plays on one of the Boomers' primary concerns (graying and aging) and marries this concern with a product that is in tune with the times* **(results are nearly instantaneous—"instant gratification" is a tremendous consumer payoff)** *plus it makes the shopping environment "relatively painless" (i.e. not embarrassing). Since, one of the most obvious signs of aging is gray hair, it's not surprising that there would be a demand for this product.*

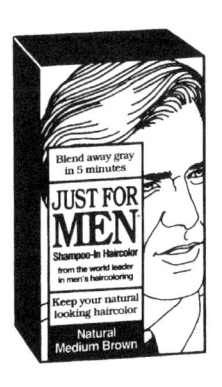

Nevertheless, companies have tried before to put forward men's hair coloring, but none had been successful. Comb steered to success by taking a page from Procter & Gamble's hugely successful Secret Deodorant "manual" ("strong enough for a man, made for a woman"). The product is marketed in the men's section, and the package clearly communicates "manly"; it also gives options in terms of coverage (light to dark) and promises to "gradually cover gray." There is little dissonance in terms of "what would people say" (as in the case of a bad fitting toupee). Although only five years old, its annual sales are close to $80 million at retail and the growth rate is still at double digits.[57]

On the surface, the remaining elements of this segment's products (hairsprays, oils, and gels) appear to offer steady but "unspectacular" growth. However, when the margin structures are examined, it's clear that these staid brands have a real consumer franchise. The fact that there has been growth at all on Vitalis, Brylcreem, Consort, and Wildroot speaks volumes to the loyalty level in men's grooming products. Thus, the aging Boomers have kept the sales on these staple products steady, while support has been virtually nonexistent over the past decade. Further, the price points have tended to be on the high side, thereby keeping the margin structure strong.

Brand awareness is the key "reason why" established men's hair preparations have been able to maintain their franchise. Considering the fact that there has been virtually no support for these businesses in the past decade, the brand awareness levels are high; brands such as Brylcreem and Vitalis still have better than fifty percent brand awareness levels. Even Vaseline Hair Tonic and Gillette's Dry Look post awareness levels in the thirties (the lack of major promotional support on these businesses is the main reason why the profit margins have remained "fat"). **This is a lesson many marketers should adhere to: Older (even eroding) franchises can be profitable if "milked" correctly.**

The above shows the difficulty of breaking into the hair preparations market—high loyalty levels coupled with strong levels of "complacency" (primarily due to a lack of "new news" on the part of manufacturers, particularly at the mass level). However, **marketers who invest in real product differentiation can realize profits (ala the experience of Combe's Just For Men).**

SUMMARY: MEN'S PERSONAL CARE MARKET

The generational themes espoused in this section are as true for men as they are for women. The promise of better, younger looking skin is as appealing to the aging male Boomer as it is to the Generation X crowd. The bottom line is that men want healthy skin and are looking for simplicity. This is particularly true in the area of shaving. Thus, products that will help make shaving easier, more comfortable, and possibly treat other conditions at the same time should do extremely well.

Chapter 15

CONCLUSION

THE OBJECT OF THIS BOOK HAS BEEN TO SHOW how successful marketers have exploited the primary attributes and behavior in beauty care marketing to put forth products, revitalize core franchises, and extend brand names. These attributes and behavior are by-products of changing lifestyles, demographics, and socioeconomic conditions. **As the year 2000 approaches, these themes—an aging population, higher per capita income households, increasing stress in the workplace, more single men and women, and Xers' depressed expectations— will exert even more influence on attitudes and behavior.** *Successful beauty care marketers will develop products and positionings that will help consumers look and feel better and that will be convenient to use.*

To develop these products, we detailed the how-to's for product development, advertising, consumer promotion, trade promotion, and distribution channels. We took to market a hypothetical facial moisturizer, called DermaSmooth, and walked through each phase of the marketing process—from concept stage to market introduction.

We also have discussed the primary consumer segments that comprise the beauty care category: the Fundamentalist, the Traditionalist, the Mature Stylist, and the Impressionist. We detailed their attitudes and behavior to distinguish their differences.

Finally, the diagram opposite this page summarizes the various types of beauty care shoppers (Lowest Price Shoppers, Mass Brand Shoppers, Smart Shoppers, Quality/Status Shoppers) and the primary consumer segments that comprise each shopper sector. Understanding this configuration is the key to successfully marketing beauty care products. These purchase motivations are universal and come into play across all beauty care categories. They will continue to do so in the future.

DON'T FORGET THE BIG IDEA

In conclusion, any single element discussed in this book is worthless without the Big Idea. Over and over again, I have tried to establish through examples and in practice that **the marketing process must start with the Big Idea.** To quote George Lois, "The Big Idea is the authentic source of communicative power." All the R&D, market and financial planning, advertising spending, and "excellence in execution" of a program at retail will go by the boards without the Big Idea.

In making the Big Idea happen, I believe that the words of hockey legend Wayne Gretzky (aka "The Great One") are the definitive source of knowledge: A reporter asked Gretzky why he is so much better at playing hockey than anybody else. He said, *"Everybody else watches where the puck is going but* **I go where I think it's going***.*"

Thinking ahead, doing it strategically, and being able to make decisions quickly is what the essence of successful beauty care marketing is all about.

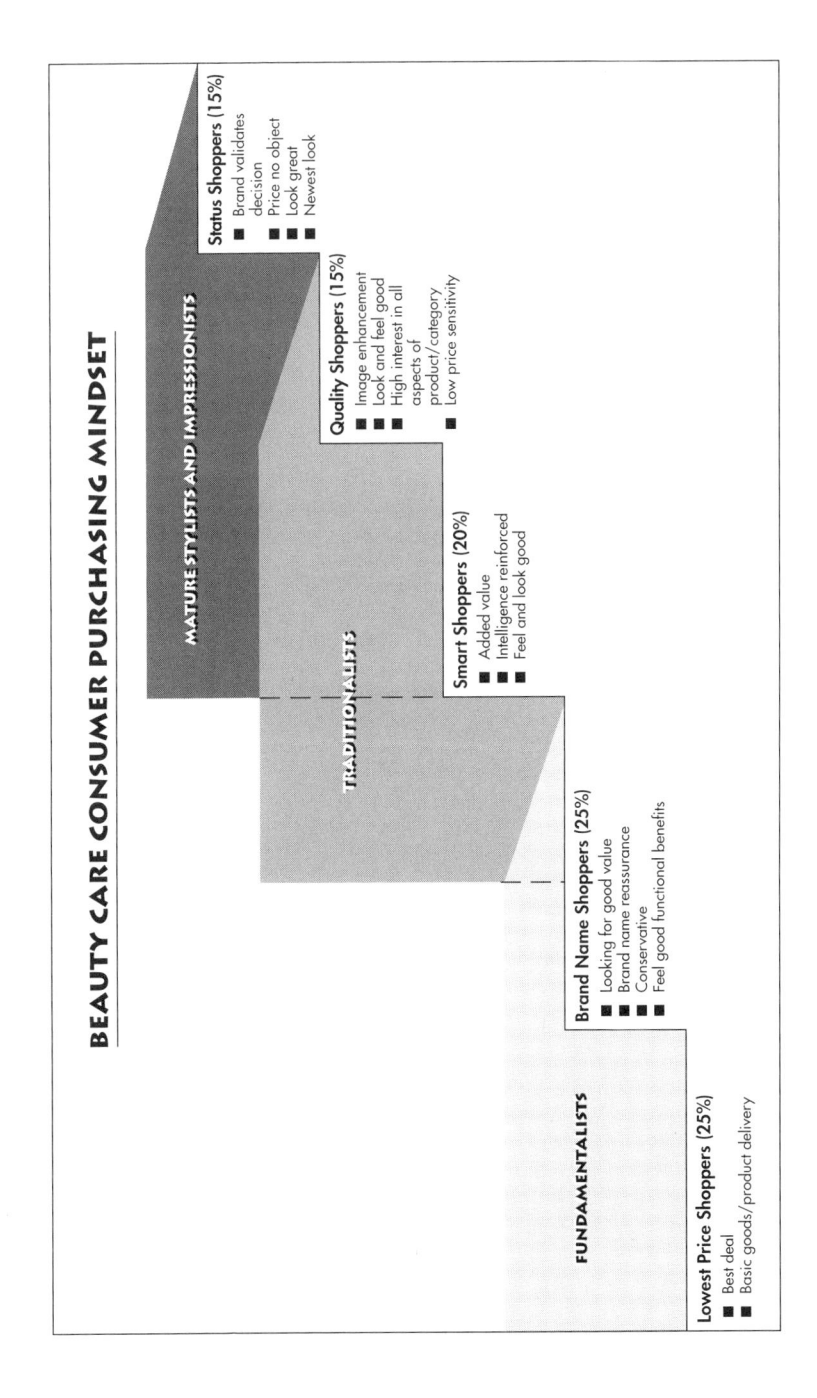

BEAUTY CARE CONSUMER PURCHASING MINDSET

MATURE STYLISTS AND IMPRESSIONISTS

Status Shoppers (15%)
- Brand validates decision
- Price no object
- Look great
- Newest look

Quality Shoppers (15%)
- Image enhancement
- Look and feel good
- High interest in all aspects of product/category
- Low price sensitivity

TRADITIONALISTS

Smart Shoppers (20%)
- Added value
- Intelligence reinforced
- Feel and look good

Brand Name Shoppers (25%)
- Looking for good value
- Brand name reassurance
- Conservative
- Feel good functional benefits

FUNDAMENTALISTS

Lowest Price Shoppers (25%)
- Best deal
- Basic goods/product delivery

Conclusion **195**

NOTES

INTRODUCTION

1. "The Beauty Top 50: A Who's Who of Cosmetics Special Report," *WWD* (Sept. 8, 1995): 1.

CHAPTER 1

1. "The Beauty Top 50: A Who's Who Of Cosmetics. Special Report," *WWD* (Sept. 8, 1995): 1.

"The Goldman Sachs 1987 Data Base," Investment Research, Personal Care Industry: 3.

"Product Marketing," *Consumer Expenditures Study* (July/August 1988).

Maria Mallory, Dan McGraw, Jill Jordan Sieder, and David Fisher, "Women On A Fast Track," *U.S. News & World Report,* Business & Technology Vol. 119, No. 18 (Nov. 6, 1995): 60.

"What's Driving Cosmetic Sales?" *Drug Store News* Vol. 17, No. 9 (June 6, 1995): 71.

Information Resources Inc., "Cosmetic and HBA Category Sales," 52 weeks ending 3/24/96.

2. Information Resources Inc., 52 weeks ending 7/14/96.

3. Bud Brewster, "50 Years of Cosmetic Color," *Cosmetics and Toiletries* Vol. 110, No. 12 (December 1995): 107.

4. Ibid.

5. Ibid.

6. "What's In A Name?" *WWD Infotracs, Second in a Series on Critical Issues,* a supplement to *WWD* (November 1995): 10.

CHAPTER 2

1. Faye Brookman, "L'Oreal-Maybelline Combo Will Give P&G A Run For Its Money," *Women's Wear Daily,* Vol. 170, No. 112 (December 15, 1995): 1.

2. Ibid.

3. "Ethnic Make-Up," *Cosmetics and Toiletries*, (December 1995).

4. Ibid.

Faye Brookman, "L'Oreal-Maybelline Combo Will Give P&G A Run For Its Money," *Women's Wear Daily*, Vol. 170, No. 112 (December 15, 1995): 1.

5. Ibid.

6. Ibid.

7. Information Resources, Inc., "IRI Economic Times & Trends," (Third Quarter 1995): 6. Criteria for success were based on an item securing at least thirty percent distribution within a two-year period.

8. Ibid.

9. Ibid.

10. Zachery Shiller, "Make It Simple," *Business Week*, September 9, 1996: 96–104.

11. "Middlescence and Beyond," International Mass Retail Association; Newspaper Association of America (1996): 2-3.

12. "Those Aging Boomers: Grayer? Sure. Slowing Down? Never. A Marketing Challenge? Absolutely!", *Business Week*, May 20, 1991: 106–112.

13. Iris Risendahl, "Skin Care Sales Reflect Consumers Concern About Aging," *Drug Topics*, Vol. 139, No. 14 (July 24, 1995): 60.

14. Susan Mitchell, *The Official Guide to the Generations*, (1st Edition 1995), 4.

15. Karen Hoppe, "The Glamour Beauty Survey: Consumers Demanding Value, Convenience, Multiple Benefits," *Drug & Cosmetic Industry*, Vol. 157, No. 4. (October 1995): 38.

16. Ibid., 38.

17. Iris Risendahl, "Skin Care Sales Reflect Consumers Concern About Aging," *Drug Topics*, Vol. 139, No. 14 (July 24, 1995): 60.

18. Ibid.

19. Susan Mitchell, *The Official Guide to the Generations*, (1st Edition 1995), 4.

20. "Middlescence and Beyond," International Mass Retail Association; Newspaper Association of America (1996): 2-3.

21. Ibid.

22. Maria Mallory, Dan McGraw, Jill Jordan Sieder, and David Fisher, "Women On A Fast Track," *U.S. News & World Report*, Business & Technology Section, Vol. 119, No. 18. (Nov. 6, 1995): 60.

23. *The Statistical Abstract of the United States 1995* (115th Edition), 465.

Susan Mitchell, *The Official Guide to the Generations*, (1st Edition 1995), 245, 249.

24. *The Statistical Abstract of the United States 1995* (115th Edition), 399.

25. Ibid.

26. Susan Mitchell, *The Official Guide to the Generations*, (1st Edition 1995), 145.

27. Ibid.

28. Iris Risendahl, "Skin Care Sales Reflect Consumers Concern About Aging," *Drug Topics*, Vol. 139, No. 14 (July 24, 1995): 60.

29. "Demographics: A View to the Future," Bush Boake Allen Inc, presented to Colgate-Palmolive Co. in 1989.

"Ethnic Makeup," *Cosmetics & Toiletries* (December 1995).

30. "Ethnic Personal Care Products Market Growth," *Minority Markets Alert* (June 1995).

31. David W. Gibson, "More Than Skin Deep; Skincare and Suncare Products; Personal Care '94," *Chemical Marketing Reporter*, Vol. 245, No. 19 (May 9, 1994): SR8.

CHAPTER 3

1. Information Resources, Inc., 52 weeks ending 4/21/96.

2. Jim Findler, "How to Beat the Odds in the New Products Game," *IRI Economic Times & Trends*, Third Quarter 1995, Information Resources Inc.: 6.

3. Ibid.

4. Cara Kagan, "Facing the Future: Mass Market Cosmetic Companies," *Woman's Wear Daily*, Special Report, Vol. 120, No. 57: S6.

5. Ibid.

6. Alexander Bid, executive director of the Ogilvy Center for Research & Development, "The Advertising/Sales Promotion Mix: A Look at the Bottom Line," speech given to the Advertising Research Foundation's 35th Annual Conference (April 10, 1989) transcript proceedings: 66-73.

7. Michael Perry, worldwide coordinator of personal care for Unilever, "Building World Class Beauty Brands," speech given to the Cosmetic Women's Executive Association (October 4, 1989).

8. Zachary Schiller, "The Sound and the Flouride," *Business Week* (Aug. 14, 1995): 48.

9. Dennis Chase, "Can Unique Selling Proposition Find Happiness in Parity World?" *Advertising Age* (September 21, 1992): 56.

10. Susan Mitchell, *The Official Guide to the Generations* (1st Edition 1995), 4.

11. Jennifer Egan, "I'm CK, You're CK," *Elle* (October 1994).

12. Carolyn J. Poppe, "A Better Mousetrap: The Secret to R&D Success," includes related article on "Increased Research and Development Spending Forecasts," *Soap Cosmetics; Chemical Specialties*, Vol. 72, No. 2 (February 1996): 21.

13. Maria Mallory, Dan McGraw, Jill Jordan Sieder, and David Fisher, "Women On A Fast Track," *U.S. News & World Report*, Vol. 119, No. 18 (November 6, 1995): 60.

14. Ibid.

15. Cara Kagan, "Facing The Future: Mass-Market Cosmetics Companies," Special Report: Color Cosmetics Industry Overview, *Women's Wear Daily*, Vol. 170, No. 57 (September 22, 1995): S6.

16. Nielsen Marketing Research, "Fifth Annual Survey of Manufacturer Trade Promotion Practices" (May 1994): 7.

17. John C. Schroer, "Ad Spending: Growing Market Share," *Harvard Business Review* Reprint 90113 (May-June 1990): 16.

18. Ibid.

19. Ibid.

20. Ibid.

21. Nielsen Marketing Research, "Fifth Annual Survey of Manufacturer Trade Promotion Practices" (May 1994): 7.

22. Stephen J. Hoch, Xavier Dreze, and Mary E. Purk, "EDLP, HI-LO and Margin Arithmetic," *Journal of Marketing* Fall 1994, Vol. 58, No.4: 16.

23. Susan Chandler, "Reinventing The Store," *Business Week* (November 27, 1995): 96.

24. Kurt Salmon Associates, "Retail Trends & Vision 2010," speech given on January 22, 1996 to the International Mass Retail Association's Fourth Annual Leadership Conference: 1.

25. Joel Benson Associates. Custom research project for Kayser-Roth conducted among 150 human resource directors of Fortune 1000 companies.

26. Susan Chandler, "Reinventing The Store," *Business Week* (November 27, 1995): 96.

27. "Store Tie-Ins Launch Green Cosmetics Line," *Public Relations Journal* (April 1991): 24.

28. Katherine Snow Smith, "Old Hyde Park to House Estee Lauder's Green Line," *Tampa Bay Business Journal*, Vol. 14, No. 18, Sec. 1: 1.

29. Ibid.

30. "Store Tie-Ins Launch Green Cosmetics Line," *Public Relations Journal* (April 1991): 24.

31. "The Origin of Cosmetics," *The Dallas Morning News* (Dec. 8, 1993).

32. Information Resources Inc., 52 Weeks Ending 6/96.

33. "What's Driving Cosmetic Sales?" *Drug Store News*, Vol. 17, No. 9 (June 26, 1995): 71. NACDS Executive Category Review & Merchandising Manual 1992.

34. Yankelovich, Skelley and White, Inc., "Monitor 1983."

35. "What's Driving Cosmetic Sales?" *Drug Store News*, Vol. 17, No. 9 (June 26, 1995): 71. NACDS Executive Category Review & Merchandising Manual 1992.

36. HTI 1995 consumer purchasing panel on legwear. Proprietary 50,000 household consumer panel prepared for the Kayser-Roth Corporation.

37. NPD panel data. Based on Kayser-Roth's 50,000 household panel of legwear shoppers.

CHAPTER 4

1. "Beauty Attitudes and Images of U.S. Women," *Glamour*, 1988.

"A National Study of Women: Beauty Product Purchasing Habits and Attitudes," *Self*, 1986 Beauty Study.

Mark Clements Research, Inc.; National Family Opinion, Inc.; SRI-VALS International; Kayser-Roth, "1994 Update: Women's Legwear Market."

2. Ian Morrison, *The Second Curve* (New York: Ballantine Books), 8.

3. Ibid., 9.

4. Ibid., 9.

CHAPTER 5

1. "Beauty Attitudes and Images of U.S. Women," a segmentation analysis developed with and for the beauty industry by *Glamour* (1988).

2. Ibid.

3. Ibid.

CHAPTERS 6–9

1. Maria Mallory, Dan McGraw, Jill Jordan Sieder, and David Fisher, "Women On A Fast Track," *U.S. News and World Report*, Vol. 119, No. 18 (November 6, 1995): 60.

2. Maria Mallory, Dan McGraw, Jill Jordan Sieder, and David Fisher, "Women On A Fast Track," *U.S. News and World Report*, Vol. 119, No. 18 (November 6, 1995): 60.

"Total Cosmetic Market: Beauty Product Marketing," Consumer Expenditure Study (July/August 1988): 11.

The Statistical Abstract of the United States 1995 (115th Edition), 492, Table 781.

3. Maria Mallory, Dan McGraw, Jill Jordan Sieder, and David Fisher, "Women On A Fast Track," *U.S. News and World Report*, Vol. 119, No. 18 (November 6, 1995): 60.

4. Information Resources, Inc., "Mass Market Cosmetic Sales," 52 weeks ending 3/24/96.

5. Cara Kagan, "Facing the Future: Mass-Market Cosmetics Companies," *Women's Wear Daily*, Special Report: Color Cosmetics Industry Overview, Vol. 170, No. 57 (September, 22, 1995): S6.

6. Ibid.

7. Information Resources Inc., "Mass Market Cosmetic Sales," 52 weeks ending 3/24/96.

8. "Long-Lasting Formulas Energize Lipstick Category," *Health and Beauty Care Executive*, Vol. 1, No. 7 (August 7, 1995): 1.

9. Ibid.

10. Ibid.

11. Information Resources Inc., "Mass Market Cosmetic Sales," 52 weeks ending 3/24/96.

12. Bud Brewster, "50 Years of Cosmetic Color," Cosmetics and Toiletries, December 1995.

13. Ibid.

14. Ibid.

15. Ibid

16. Cara Kagan, "Facing the Future: Mass-Market Cosmetics Companies," Special Report: Color Cosmetics Industry Overview, *Women's Wear Daily*, Vol. 170, No. 57 (September 22, 1995).

17. "The Beauty Top 50: A Who's Who of Cosmetics," *Women's Wear Daily*, Special Report (September 8, 1995):1.

Investment Research, Personal Care Industry. The Goldman Sachs 1987 Data Base, 3.

"Consumer Expenditures Study: Product Marketing," *U.S. News and World Report*, Business and Technology (July/August 1988).

Maria Mallory, Dan McGraw, Jill Jordan Sieder, and David Fisher, "Women On A Fast Track," *U.S. News and World Report*, Vol. 119, No. 18 (November 6, 1995): 60.

"What's Driving Cosmetic Sales?" *Drug Store News*, Vol. 17, No. 9 (June 6, 1995): 71.

Information Resources Inc., "Cosmetic and HBA Category Sales," 52 weeks ending 3/24/96.

18. Ibid.

19. Ibid.

20. "U.S. Hand and Body Lotion Market," Report for Colgate-Palmolive (February 1991).

21. "Beauty Attitudes and Images of U.S. Women," *Glamour* (1988).

22. "The Beauty Top 50: A Who's Who of Cosmetics," *Women's Wear Daily*, Special Report (September 8, 1995):1.

Investment Research, Personal Care Industry. The Goldman Sachs 1987 Data Base, 3.

"Consumer Expenditures Study: Product Marketing," *U.S. News and World Report*, Business and Technology (July/August 1988).

Maria Mallory, Dan McGraw, Jill Jordan Sieder, and David Fisher, "Women On A Fast Track," *U.S. News and World Report*, Vol. 119, No. 18 (November 6, 1995): 60.

"What's Driving Cosmetic Sales?" *Drug Store News*, Vol. 17, No. 9 (June 6, 1995): 71.

Information Resources Inc., "Cosmetic and HBA Category Sales," 52 weeks ending 3/24/96.

23. "Beauty Attitudes and Images of U.S. Women," *Glamour* (1988).

24. David W. Gibson, "More Than Skin Deep," *Chemical Marketing Reporter*, Vol. 245, No. 19 (May 9, 1994): SR8.

25. Ibid.

26. "The Beauty Top 50: A Who's Who of Cosmetics," *Women's Wear Daily*, Special Report (September 8, 1995):1.

27. David W. Gibson, "More Than Skin Deep," *Chemical Marketing Reporter*, Vol. 245, No. 19 (May 9, 1994): SR8.

28. "The Beauty Top 50: A Who's Who of Cosmetics," *Women's Wear Daily*, Special Report (September 8, 1995):1.

Investment Research, Personal Care Industry. The Goldman Sachs 1987 Data Base, 3.

"Consumer Expenditures Study: Product Marketing," *U.S. News and World Report*, Business and Technology (July/August 1988).

Maria Mallory, Dan McGraw, Jill Jordan Sieder, and David Fisher, "Women On A Fast Track," *U.S. News and World Report*, Vol. 119, No. 18 (November 6, 1995): 60.

"What's Driving Cosmetic Sales?" *Drug Store News*, Vol. 17, No. 9 (June 6, 1995): 71.

Information Resources Inc., "Cosmetic and HBA Category Sales," 52 weeks ending 3/24/96.

29. *1992 NACDS Executive Category Review and Merchandising Manual*, 233.

30. Investment Research, Personal Care Industry. The Goldman Sachs 1987 Data Base, 3.

"Consumer Expenditures Study: Product Marketing," *U.S. News and World Report*, Business and Technology (July/August 1988).

Maria Mallory, Dan McGraw, Jill Jordan Sieder, and David Fisher, "Women On A Fast Track," *U.S. News and World Report*, Vol. 119, No. 18 (November 6, 1995): 60.

"What's Driving Cosmetic Sales?" *Drug Store News*, Vol. 17, No. 9 (June 6, 1995): 71.

Information Resources Inc., "Cosmetic and HBA Category Sales," 52 weeks ending 3/24/96.

31. "Jergens Launches Shower Active Moisturizer," PR Newswire (November 14, 1995).

32. "Bath Additives—Liquid," *Drug Store News*, Vol. 17, No. 9 (June 26, 1995): 172.

"Jergens Launches Shower Active Moisturizer," PR Newswire (November 14, 1995).

"Beauty Attitudes and Images of U.S. Women," *Glamour* (1988).

33. Ibid.

34. Carolyn J. Poppe, "A Better Mousetrap: The Secrets to R&D Success," *Soap-Cosmetics-Chemical Specialties*, Vol. 72, No. 2 (February 1996): 21.

35. "Jergens Launches Shower Active Moisturizer," PR Newswire (November 14, 1995).

36. Shelley M. Colwell, "Never Say Dye—Hair Colorants Are On The Rise," *Soap-Cosmetics-Chemical Specialties*, Vol. 70, No. 10 (October 1994): 20.

37. Victoria Wurdinger, "Hair Care Report," *Drug and Cosmetic Industry*, Vol. 158, No. 4 (April 1996): 24.

38. Margaret Vogel, "The Hair Care Market," *HAPPI* (*Household and Personal Products Industry*) (November 1987): 48.

39. Hair Care, Nielsen Marketing Research's National Electronic Household Panel, *Drug Store News*, Special Section "Consumer Shopping Habits," Vol. 16, No. 10 (June 27, 1994): 59.

40. Lisa Kintish, "Shampoos Get Specific," *Soap-Cosmetics-Chemical Specialties*, Vol. 71, No. 10 (October 1995): 20.

41. Victoria Wurdinger, "Hair Care Additives: From the Rain Forest to the Test Tube the Focus Is on Efficacy," *Drug and Cosmetic Industry*, Vol. 157, No. 6 (December 1995): 20.

42. Ibid.

43. Ibid.

44. Information Resources Inc., 52 weeks ending 5/27/94, 5/27/95, 5/27/96.

45. Shelley M. Colwell, "Never Say Dye—Hair Colorants Are On The Rise," *Soap-Cosmetics-Chemical Specialties*, Vol. 70, No. 10 (October 1994): 20.

46. Ibid.

47. Ibid.

48. Ibid.

49. Ibid.

50. Ibid.

51. Margaret Vogel, "The Hair Care Market," *HAPPI* (*Household and Personal Products Industry*) (November 1987): 48.

52. William Myers, "Cosmair Makes A Name For Itself," *New York Times*, (May 12, 1985): 25.

53. Ibid.

54. Margaret Vogel, "The Hair Care Market," *HAPPI* (*Household and Personal Products Industry*) (November 1987): 48.

55. "The Beauty Top 50: A Who's Who of Cosmetics," *Women's Wear Daily*, Special Report (September 8, 1995):1.

Investment Research, Personal Care Industry. The Goldman Sachs 1987 Data Base, 3.

"Consumer Expenditures Study: Product Marketing," *U.S. News and World Report*, Business and Technology (July/August 1988).

Maria Mallory, Dan McGraw, Jill Jordan Sieder, and David Fisher, "Women On A Fast Track," *U.S. News and World Report*, Vol. 119, No. 18 (November 6, 1995): 60.

"What's Driving Cosmetic Sales?" *Drug Store News*, Vol. 17, No. 9 (June 6, 1995): 71.

Information Resources Inc., "Cosmetic and HBA Category Sales," 52 weeks ending 3/24/96.

56. Barabar Pash, "Scent-Sational," *Baltimore Jewish Times*, Vol. 226, No. 6 (December 8, 1995): G15.

57. Alice Rawsthorn, "Marketing Fragrance Evolves Into Tooth and Nail Competition," *The Financial Post* (December 19, 1995): Section I.

58. Judith Gubbay, "How to Spend It," *The Financial Times* (November 25, 1995).

59. Meg Carter, "Scent of a Woman," *The Guardian* (September 1, 1994).

60. Alice Rawsthorn, "A Smelling Salt for the Market," *Financial Times*, Marketing and Advertising Section (March 11, 1993): 19.

61. Ibid.

62. Maxine Wilkie, "Names That Smell," *American Demographics* (August 1995): 48.

63. Ibid.

64. Ibid.

65. Meg Carter, "Scent of a Woman: Will We Wear Unisex Perfume?" *The Guardian* (September 1, 1994): 79.

66. Ibid.

CHAPTER 11–13

1. David M. Zeitlin and Richard A. Westwood, "Measuring Emotional Response," *Journal of Advertising Research* (October/November 1986): 34.

2. Ibid.

3. Michael Prone, "Package design has stronger ROI potential than many believe," *Marketing News* (October 11, 1993): 13.

4. Carolyn J. Poppe, "A better mousetrap: the secrets to R&D success," *Soap Cosmetics Chemical Specialties*, Vol. 72, No. 2 (February 1996): 21.

5. Ibid.

6. Ibid.

7. Ibid.

8. Information Resources, Inc., 52 weeks ending 5/19/96.

9. Nielsen Fifth Annual Survey of Manufacturer Trade Promotion Practices, Nielsen Marketing Research (May 1994).

10. "Beauty's New Face: Mass Merchandising of Cosmetics," *Discount Store News*, Vol. 34, No. 12 (June 19, 1995): A22.

11. Ibid.

12. Ibid.

13. Ibid

CHAPTER 14

1. Judith Langer, "A Woman Is Still A Woman, But A Man Now Has His Doubts," *Marketing News*, Qualitative Market Research/The Langer Report, (August 28, 1987).

2. The Esquire Report, "The American Man In Transition," prepared in Conjunction with Batelle Human Research Centers, Seattle, Washington (1988): 12.

3. Ibid.

Statistical Abstract of the United States 1995, 115th Edition, 104.

4. The Esquire Report, "The American Man In Transition," prepared in Conjunction with Batelle Human Research Centers, Seattle, Washington (1988): 12.

Susan Mitchell, *The Official Guide to the Generations*, 1st Edition (1995), 145.

5. Shelley M. Colwell, "Men's Toiletries Take Off," *Soap Cosmetics Chemical Specialties*, Vol. 70, No. 12 (December 1994): 30.

6. "Men's Care Markets To Top $9 Billion By 2000, Growing At 4% Per Year," 1995 Business Wire, Inc., Dateline: Mountain View, California (April 29, 1995).

7. Ibid.

8. *Statistical Abstract of the United States 1995*, 115th Edition, 17, Table #17.

9. Ibid.

10. Laura Zinn, with Christopher Power, Dori Jones, Alice Z. Cuneo, and David Ross, "Move Over Boomers, the Busters Are Here—And They're Angry," *Business Week* (December 14, 1992): 74.

11. Ibid., 77.

12. Susan Mitchell, *The Official Guide to the Generations*, 1st Edition (1995), 173.

13. Laura Zinn, with Christopher Power, Dori Jones, Alice Z. Cuneo, and David Ross, "Move Over Boomers, the Busters Are Here—And They're Angry," *Business Week* (December 14, 1992): 74.

14 *Statistical Abstract of the United States 1995*, 115th Edition, 477, Table #737.

15. Shelley M. Colwell, "Men's Toiletries Take Off," *Soap Cosmetics Chemical Specialties*, Vol. 70, No. 12 (December 1994): 30.

16. *Statistical Abstract of the United States 1995*, 115th Edition, 474, Table #731.

17. Shelley M. Colwell, "Men's Toiletries Take Off," *Soap Cosmetics Chemical Specialties*, Vol. 70, No. 12 (December 1994): 30.

18. "Men's Care Markets To Top $9 Billion By 2000, Growing At 4% Per Year," 1995 Business Wire, Inc., Dateline: Mountain View, California (April 29, 1995).

19. Ibid.

20. Carolyn J. Poppe, "The Tide Turns For Men's Products," *Soap Cosmetics Chemical Specialties*, Vol. 71, No. 12 (December 1995): 18.

21. Ruth La Ferla, "Putting on a Renewed Face," *New York Times Magazine* (October 26, 1986): 72.

22. Ibid.

23. Colgate Palmolive, "Body Care Habits & Practices," 600 Household Diary Panel conducted in March 1989 and July 1989, Appendix, 4.

24. Ibid., Appendix, 7.

25. Ibid., Main Report, 82.

26. Ibid.

27. Ibid., Appendix, 13.

28. Information Resources, Inc., 52 weeks ending 5/19/96.

29. Ibid.

30. "Shaving Segment Among The Strongest In Toiletries," *Chain Drug Review* (Vol. 18, No. 3): 38.

31. Ibid.

32. Ibid.

33. Lisa I. Fried, "What's Hot In '96. HBC: Toiletries," *Drug Store News* (Vol. 18, No.1): 19.

34. Ibid.

35. Mark Maremont with Paula Dwyer, "How Gillette Is Honing Its Edge," *Business Week* (September 28, 1992): 60.

36. Pam Weisz, "The Razor's Edge," *Brandweek* (April 24, 1995): 26.

37. Ibid.

38. Ibid.

39. Ibid.

40. "Innovations Spur Shaving Category," *Chain Drug Review* (Vol. 16, No. 19): 22.

41. Ibid.

42. Ibid.

43. "Introducing Skin Maintenance For Men From Paco Rabanne," *New York Times Magazine* (November 4, 1984): 79.

44. Information Resources, Inc., 52 weeks ending 2/25/96.

45. Norma Sexton, "Gwps and Pwps Losing Edge As Promotional Tools," *Advertising Age* (March 2, 1987).

46. "New Launches Expected To Stir Sales In Men's Scents," *Health & Beauty Care Executive*, Vol. 1, No. 42 (April 15, 1996): 1.

47. Ibid.

48. Ibid.

49. Ibid.

50. "Retailers: Solid Sales In Men's Grooming Category," *Health & Beauty Care Executive*, Vol. 1, No. 36 (March 4, 1996): 1.

51. Sean Mehegan, "Williams Sets $10M For Aqua Vela Intros," *Brandweek* (May 6, 1996): 3.

52. Ibid.

53. Shelley M. Colwell, "Men's Toiletries Take Off," *Soap Cosmetics Chemical Specialties*, Vol. 70, No. 12 (December 1994): 30.

54. Lisa I. Fried, "What's Hot In '96. HBC: Toiletries," *Drug Store News* (Vol. 18, No.1): 19.

55. Information Resources, Inc., 52 weeks ending 5/19/95.

56. Information Resources, Inc., 52 weeks ending 5/16/96.

57. "Retailers: Solid Sales In Men's Grooming Category," *Health & Beauty Care Executive*, Vol. 1, No. 36 (March 4, 1996): 4.

INDEX

absence of negatives 94
acquisitions
   in beauty care 26–27
advertising 48–49, 51, 60–61, 109
   components of 159
   melding emotion and function 161
   print vs. television 155, 160
   selecting the medium 160
   testing service companies 162
   vs. promotion 171
Almay 27
Alpha Hydroxy Acid products 110
anti-aging products 100, 110, 111
anti-wrinkling products 110
Aqua Velva 187
   extending brands 188
Armani, Georgio 140
awareness 150

bath and liquid body cleanser
   market dynamics 116
   marketing 116–17
beauty care market 19
   segments 73–75
   United States 26
beauty care marketing
   elements for success 20
   forces driving 25
   future outlook 72
   requirements for success 41
beauty care products
   active 37

cosmetic 37
   therapeutic 37, 38
beauty regimen 84, 99, 179
Big Idea 40, 51–54
   developing 144
biotechnology 46–48
Boomers 112, 127
   and retarding the aging process 100
   marketing to 30–32
   men and aging 176
   singlehood and 173
brand awareness 190
brand positioning
   components of 22–24
   problem/solution 84
   scientific 47
brands 21–22
   definition of 24
   extending 188
   focusing on 20
   importance in beauty care 42
   niche 60
   prestige 47, 63
      hair care 120
   refreshing 55, 94
   reinventing 56–57
   store vs. beauty 20
Brewster, Bud 97

Calvin Klein 52–54
   CK one 33, 53–54, 186
   Obsession 186

Campinell, Joseph 134
Canoe 187
Carter, Linda 102
case study
  !ex'cla-ma'tion 87
  Calvin Klein
    CK one 53–54
  Clairol
    Ultress 86–87
  Colgate
    Mennen Deodorant 180–81
  Colgate Palmolive 43–44
  Comb
    Just for Men Hair Coloring 188
  Estee Lauder
    Origins 64–66
  Gillette
    Sensor for Women 182
  Head & Shoulders 81
  Longing 87
  Maybelline
    Nail Enamel 79
  Paco Rabanne
    Skin Maintenance for Men 184
  Pierre Cardin 186–87
  Ponds
    Age Defying System 84
  Procter & Gamble
    Oil of Olay 45–46
  Revlon
    ColorStay Lipstick 57–58
  Unilever
    Mentadent Toothpaste 50–51
casual dress 40
effects on beauty care marketing 63
celebrity spokespeople 98
Chanel 140
  Chanel No. 5 140
Chanel, Gabrielle 140
Chesebrough-Ponds 27
  Aziza Nail Polish Pen 98
  Ponds 27
  Rave 27, 131–33
  Vaseline 27

Clairol
  hair coloring products 130
  Ultress 86–87
class marketers 96
Colgate Palmolive
  Facial Bar Soap 43–44
  Mennen Deodorant 180–81
  on product development 166
Comb
  hair coloring for men 188
communication 159, 164
concept 144
  development 144–46
  evaluation 146–47
  white care 145
consumer behavior
  changing 108
Copeland, Douglas 33
copy strategy 52, 157–58
core franchises
  refreshing 54–58
cosmetics 19, 26
  ethnic 27
  market dynamics 95
  marketing 95–104
  price of entry 93
  primary segments 95
Coty
  Hold It 99
  Raw Vanilla 186
  Stetson 187
couponing 170, 171
Cover Girl 27
  Balanced Complexion Liquid Makeup 100
Crawford, Joan 102
Curtis, Jamie Lee 109

Delagar
  Gender One 186
deo-colognes 40
distribution 150
divorce 35, 173, 177
Dressler, Fran 109
Dwyer, Kathy 57

eligible population base 149
Elka 97
Estee Lauder 64
   Origins 64–66
   Thigh Zone Body Streamlining
      Complex 109
Eternity 186
ethnic market
   understanding 36–37
everyday fair price 66
everyday low price (EDLP) 61–62
!ex'cla-ma'tion 87
eye makeup
   marketing 101–104
   positioning examples 102–104

Faberge
   Brut 187, 188
facial cleanser
   market dynamics 112
   marketing 112–13
   positioning examples 113
facial makeup
   marketing 100–101
   positioning examples 100–101
   primary benefits 100
facial moisturizer
   market dynamics 110
   marketing 110–12
   positioning examples 111–12
   price of entry 110
fair price 70
fragrance 19, 26, 46
   celebrity themes 39
   knock-off designer 39
   pricing in market 39
frequency 158–59
Fundamentalist 73, 75, 77–79

Generation Xers
   52, 101, 127, 135, 141
   difficulty of marketing to men 176
   lifestyles and income 35
   marketing to 32–37
   generational marketing 22–23,
      30–34, 64, 188

Generation Xers 32
   older Boomers 30–31
   younger Boomers 31–32
Gillette
   Sensor for Women 182–83
   Sensor Razor 182
Gravity 185
green marketing 64
Griffith, Melanie 100

hair care 19, 26
   future of 126
   market dynamics 119
   marketing 119–35
   prestige brands 120
   segmentation 121
   temporary hair coloring 56
   usage 120
hair coloring products 127–31
   positioning examples 130
hairspray
   reinventing 134
Hamilton, Carol 130, 134
hand and body lotion
   failure of secondary positioning
      107
   market dynamics 106
   marketing 106–10
   positioning examples 107–10
Hawaiian Tropics 114
Hay, Heather 183
Hilfiger, Tommy 141

Impressionist 73, 85–90, 101, 135
in-store demonstrations 88
in-store sampling 85
income 177, 178
   buying power and personal care
      products 34–35
   changes in purchasing habits 39
initial gross profit 59

Jean Phillippe
   A Man and A Woman 186
Jergens
   Body Shampoo 116

Shower Active 116–17
Jovan 187

Lachman, Charles 97
Lamar, Hedy 102
lifestyles
   changing trends in men's 173–74, 177–78
   understanding trends in 53
liposomes 111
lipstick 97
   market dynamics 99
   marketing 99–100
   positioning examples 99–100
   primary benefits 99
Lois, George 51
Longing 87
L'Oreal 95, 161
   Color Endure Lipstick 99
   Freehold Mousse 134
   Gio 139–40
   hair care products 126
   hair coloring products 130
   Plenitude 111
   purchase of Maybelline 26–27
   Revitalift Firming Creme 111
   Voluminous Waterproof Mascara 102
Lubriderm 161

Mandor, Tanya 172
Marcus, Raulee 44
market fragmentation 24, 28–29, 101
   avoiding pitfalls in 38–40
market segmentation 24
market share 70
   growing 60–61
Mary Kay
   Skin Revival System 112
mass marketers 96
Matrix Essentials 127
Mature Stylist 73, 75, 82–85, 100, 111
Max Factor 27
Maybelline 95

Alpha Hydroxy Intensive Night Creme 112
   Lash by Lash Mascara 102
   Nail Enamel 79
   purchase by L'Oreal 26–27
   Revitalizing Makeup 101
McDonald, Camille 188
McGreevy, Rebecca C. 65
mega-branding 42–46
men's personal care market 40, 173–91
   body cleansers 179–80
   deodorants 180–81
   fragrances 185–88
      unisex 186
   hair grooming products 188–90
   increase in male-oriented sections in stores 178
   market dynamics 175
   primary drivers 175
   self-confident themes in 173
   shaving products 182–84
   unisex products 177
mergers. *See* acquisitions
Morrison, Ian 72
Moss, Kate 54
Mottus, Alan 135
Mozingo, Jim 66

nail enamel
   introduction of color to cosmetics 96
   market dynamics 96
   marketing 96–98
   positioning examples 98
   primary benefits 98
Navy For Men 187
Nivea
   Visage Optimale Cumulative Care Creme 111
Noxema 113

Opal, Black 183

packaging 133
   brief 163

CK one 141
development 163–65
testing 164–65
Paco Rabanne
Skin Maintenance for Men 184
Parfum de Coeur
U 186
Perry, Mike 49
persuasion 160
Phillips, Sue G. 179
Pierre Cardin 186–87
point of difference 23
Ponds Age Defying System 84
Preferred Stock 187
price of entry 23, 73
advertising 49
anti-aging properties 100, 111
benefits 93–94
hand and body lotion benefits 107
improving combination skin 101
long lasting 55
nourishment and cleaning 113
price/value equation 63, 64, 70
establishing the right price 66–70
rethinking in the 1970s and 1980s 67–68
pricing 100
CK one 141
EDLP 61–63
high-low 62
in beauty care marketing 54
primary drivers 94
Procter & Gamble 26, 27, 61
and fragmentation marketing 29
and mega-branding 45–46
Cover Girl 95
Crest Toothpaste 29
Head & Shoulders 29, 81
Oil of Olay 45–46, 113
Old Spice 187, 188
Pert 55
Wondra 107–109
product development 165–66
influence of global marketplace on 166

product differentiation 54
product introduction 169–72
working with retailers 171–72
product positioning 21–22
category drivers 93–94
eye makeup 102–104
facial cleanser 113
facial makeup 100–101
facial moisturizer 111–12
hair coloring products 130
hand and body lotion 107–10
in men's fragrances 185
lipstick 99–100
nail enamel 98
problem/solution 109
shampoo and conditioner 126–27
sun care 114
women's fragrance 139–41
product proliferation 28, 38, 165
product sampling
84, 88, 111, 170, 172
product testing 167
blind 167–68
identified product 168
promotion 48–49, 170
vs. advertising 171
promotional sales 88
purchase cycle 151
purchase interest 149

Quinn, Cindy 171

Ralph Lauren
Polo 186, 188
reach 158–59
recall 159, 164
research and development 38, 55
importance in product development 165
retention level 151
Revlon 22, 27, 95, 98, 99
Age Defying Makeup 100
ColorStay Lipstick 55–58, 99
reinventing 56
working with retailers 171–72
Revson, Charles 22, 97

Rossi, Ron 182

secondary drivers 94
shampoo and conditioner
   natural 127
   positioning examples 126–27
share of voice 60
Sheasby, Robert 188
Shields, Brooke 54
Shroer, James 60
skin care 19, 26
   market dynamics 105
Smith, Jack 134
St. Ives
   Vanilla and Honey Facial Wash 113
styling aids 131–35
   gels 135
   hairspray 131–34
   mousses 134–35
sun care
   market dynamics 114
   marketing 114–16
   positioning examples 114

technology 102, 116
   influence on men's personal care market 179
   piggybacking to launch gender specific products 182
   transference of 99
television show sponsorship 98
testing, hypoallergenic 102
Tobias, Andrew 22
tommy 185
Tommy Girl 141
total trial level 150
trade allowances 59
trade class
   deep discounters 68
   department store 63–64
   drug store 67
   food store 66
   food-drug-mass 61–63
   going from class to mass 186–88
   mass merchandiser 69–70
Traditionalist 73, 80–82
Trial & Repeat model 147–56
   internal financial proposition 153–55
   repeat components 151–52
   trial components 149–50
   Year 1 Consumer Business Opportunity 152–53
Turlington, Christy 102
Turner, Tina 109

Unilever 27, 49
   Impulse 40
   Mentadent Toothpaste 50–51
   Ponds Age Defying Moisturizer 112
   Ponds Cold Cream 55
   Vaseline Intensive Care Lotion 44–45, 107
   Vaseline Petroleum Jelly 55
unique selling proposition 23

visibility 164

Ward, Sela 109
Westwood, Richard 161
Williams, T.L. 102
women's fragrance
   and fashion 140
   market dynamics 137
   marketing 137–41
   positioning examples 139–41
   prestige 140
   usage 139
working women
   increasing in the work force 35

Zeitlin, David 161

ABOUT PINNACLE MARKETING MANAGEMENT

Pinnacle Marketing Management is a world class business consulting organization. It is a company composed of marketing information resource specialists who provide clients with a consistent process for understanding consumer behavior and attitudes in order to achieve profitable growth. Bill Koslowe, the author of *Beauty and the Beastly Market: Taming Uncertainties in Marketing Beauty Products*, is its president.

Pinnacle Marketing Management helps clients identify leverageable functional and emotional drivers across specific products and services. It details the competitive environment and the rules necessary to compete. This assures that the end goal will be both financial goal optimization and product/consumer bundle optimization. This positioning of consumer dynamics with financial plan attainment is what separates Pinnacle Marketing Management from other organizations.

To learn more about Pinnacle Marketing Management, call or write to:

Bill Koslowe
Pinnacle Marketing Management
Suite 465 Nationsbank Plaza
Winston-Salem, NC 27101-3915
Telephone: 336-856-8602
Fax: 336-856-8602
E-mail: billkos@aol.com

ABOUT THE AUTHOR

Bill Koslowe is president of Pinnacle Marketing Management. He has worked with major corporations on strategy development, forecasting, and market research. He is well versed in the marketing dynamics of North America, Western Europe, Latin America, the Far East, and Africa. He has specifically conducted studies in more than fifteen diverse markets including the United States, Canada, Mexico, Venezuela, Brazil, Italy, Germany, France, England, the Philippines, and Kenya. His client list and organzations he has worked with include Canadaigua Wine, Chesebrough-Ponds, Inc., Colgate-Palmolive, DuPont, Faberge, General Foods, Kayser-Roth, and Rexall Sundown, Inc.

He received his BBA from Pace University and his MBA from the University of New Mexico. Pinnacle Marketing Management has offices in Greensboro, North Carolina, and New York City.